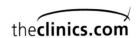

HAND CLINICS

Hand Arthritis

GUEST EDITOR
Matthew M. Tomaino, MD, MBA

May 2006 • Volume 22 • Number 2

SAUNDERS

An Imprint of Elsevier, Inc.
PHILADELPHIA   LONDON   TORONTO   MONTREAL   SYDNEY   TOKYO

W.B. SAUNDERS COMPANY

A Division of Elsevier Inc.

1600 John F. Kennedy Blvd. • Suite 1800 • Philadelphia, Pennsylvania 19103

http://www.theclinics.com

HAND CLINICS
May 2006
Editor: Debora Dellapena

Volume 22, Number 2
ISSN 0749-0712
ISBN 1-4160-3507-9

The ideas and opinions expressed in *Hand Clinics* do not necessarily reflect those of the Publisher. The Publisher does not assume any responsibility for any injury and/or damage to persons or property arising out of or related to any use of the material contained in this periodical. The reader is advised to check the appropriate medical literature and the product information provided by the manufacturer of each drug to be administered to verify the dosage, the method and duration of administration, or contraindications. It is the responsibility of the treating physician or other health care professional, relying on independent experience and knowledge of the patient, to determine drug dosages and the best treatment for the patient. Mention of any product in this issue should not be construed as endorsement by the contributors, editors, or the Publisher of the product or manufacturers' claims.

Hand Clinics (ISSN 0749-0712) is published quarterly by W.B. Saunders, 360 Park Avenue South, New York, NY 10010-1710. Months of publication are February, May, August, and November. Business and Editorial Offices: 1600 John F. Kennedy Blvd., Suite 1800, Philadelphia, PA 19103-2899. Accounting and Circulation Offices: 6277 Sea Harbor Drive, Orlando, FL 32887-4800. Periodicals postage paid at New York, NY, and additional mailing offices. Subscription price is $215.00 per year (U.S. individuals), $335.00 per year (U.S. institutions), $110.00 per year (US students), $245.00 per year (Canadian individuals), $375.00 per year (Canadian institutions), $135.00 (Canadian students), $275.00 per year (international individuals), $375.00 per year (international institutions), and $135.00 per year (international students). Foreign air speed delivery is included in all *Clinics* subscription prices. All prices are subject to change without notice. POSTMASTER: Send address changes to *Hand Clinics*, Elsevier Periodicals Customer Service, 6277 Sea Harbor Drive, Orlando, FL 32887-4800. **Customer Service: 1-800-654-2452 (US). From outside the US, call 1-407-345-4000. E-mail: hhspcs@harcourt.com.**

Reprints. For copies of 100 or more, of articles in this publication, please contact the Commercial Rights Department, Elsevier Inc., 360 Park Avenue South, New York, NY 10010-1710. Tel: (212) 633-3813, Fax: (212) 462-1935, e-mail: reprints@elsevier.com.

Hand Clinics is covered in *Index Medicus, Current Contents/Clinical Medicine, EMBASE/Excerpta Medica,* and *ISI/BIOMED.*

Printed in the United States of America.

GUEST EDITOR

MATTHEW M. TOMAINO, MD, MBA, Professor of Orthopaedics; Chief, Division of Hand, Shoulder, and Elbow Surgery; Director of Hand and Upper Extremity Fellowship; University of Rochester Medical Center, Rochester, New York

CONTRIBUTORS

ALEJANDRO BADIA, MD, FACS, Hand and Upper Extremity Surgeon, Miami Hand Center; Chief of Hand Surgery, Baptist Hospital of Miami; Director, Small Joint Arthroscopy, DaVinci Learning Center, Miami, Florida

ROBERT D. BECKENBAUGH, MD, Professor, Department of Orthopedic Surgery, Mayo Clinic College of Medicine, Rochester, Minnesota

CHARLES S. DAY, MD, MBA, Chief, Orthopaedic Hand and Upper Extremity Surgery, Department of Orthopaedic Surgery, Beth Israel Deaconess Medical Center; Assistant Professor, Harvard Medical School, Boston, Massachusetts

THOMAS T. DOVAN, MD, Orthopaedic and Sports Medicine Center, Rome, Georgia

STEVEN Z. GLICKEL, MD, Associate Clinical Professor of Orthopedic Surgery, Columbia University College of Physicians and Surgeons; Director, Hand Surgery Service, St. Luke's-Roosevelt Hospital Center, New York, New York

CHARLES A. GOLDFARB, MD, Assistant Professor, Department of Orthopaedic Surgery, Washington University School of Medicine at Barnes-Jewish Hospital, St. Louis, Missouri

SALIL GUPTA, MD, Clinical Assistant Professor of Orthopaedic Surgery, New York University School of Medicine, University Place Orthopaedic Surgery, New York, New York

KIRSTEN B. HORMEL, RN, Department of Orthopedic Surgery, Mayo Clinic College of Medicine, Rochester, Minnesota

THOMAS R. HUNT, III, MD, John D. Sherrill Professor of Surgery; Director, Division of Orthopaedic Surgery, The University of Alabama, Birmingham School of Medicine, Birmingham, Alabama

MICHAEL LEIT, MD, Clinical Assistant Professor, University of Rochester Medical Center, Rochester, New York

JOHN D. MAHONEY, MD, Clinical Instructor, Combined Orthopaedic and Plastic Surgery Hand Service, University of California, Los Angeles, Los Angeles, California

ROY A. MEALS, MD, Clinical Professor of Orthopaedic Surgery, Combined Orthopaedic and Plastic Surgery Hand Service, University of California, Los Angeles, Los Angeles, California

STEVEN L. MORAN, MD, Associate Professor, Division of Plastic Surgery and Department of Orthopedic Surgery, Mayo Clinic College of Medicine, Rochester, Minnesota

PETER M. MURRAY, MD, Associate Professor, Department of Orthopaedic Surgery, Mayo Clinic College of Medicine, Rochester, Minnesota; Consultant, Department of Orthopaedic Surgery; Chair, Division of Education, Mayo Clinic, Jacksonville, Florida

WENDY PARKER, MD, PhD, Hand Fellow, Department of Orthopedic Surgery, Mayo Clinic College of Medicine, Rochester, Minnesota

MIGUEL A. RAMIREZ, BS, Doris Duke Fellow, Harvard Medical School; Department of Orthopaedic Surgery, Beth Israel Deaconess Medical Center, Boston, Massachusetts

MARCO RIZZO, MD, Assistant Professor, Department of Orthopedic Surgery, Mayo Clinic College of Medicine, Rochester, Minnesota

MATTHEW M. TOMAINO, MD, MBA, Professor of Orthopaedics; Chief, Division of Hand, Shoulder, and Elbow Surgery; Director of Hand and Upper Extremity Fellowship; University of Rochester Medical Center, Rochester, New York

CONTENTS

This article describes the rationale and results of a "biomechanical" strategy to restore trapeziometacarpal (TM) stability when symptomatic Eaton Stage I disease exists. Though the author has performed TM arthroscopy, synovectomy, and capsular shrinkage for such cases in 10 patients, the author has been dissatisfied with the outcomes, particularly pain relief. The author currently relies exclusively on extension osteotomy as treatment for this subset of patients. Thumb metacarpal extension osteotomy remains an effective treatment alternative for the hypermobile TM joint consistent with Eaton Stage I disease. This procedure alters forces, shifts load away from the volar compartment, and further engages the dorsoradial ligament. Clinical outcomes are favorable, and no bridges are burned should arthritic changes develop in the future.

Volar ligament reconstruction uses half of the flexor carpi radialis tendon passed through a gouge hole in the base of the thumb metacarpal to substitute for an acute or chronically lax anterior oblique ligament of the thumb carpometacarpal joint. The configuration of the reconstruction functionally substitutes for the dorsoradial ligament as well. The technique has changed little since its description in 1973. When the procedure is done for patients who have Stage I or early Stage II disease, excellent to good results can be expected in upwards of 90% of patients.

Indications for arthroscopy of the trapeziometacarpal joint of the thumb remain poorly understood. Arthroscopic assessment of the carpometacarpal joint allows direct visualization of all components of the joint, including synovium, articular surfaces, ligaments, and the joint capsule. It also allows for the extent of joint pathology to be evaluated and staged with intraoperative management decisions made based on this information. A proposed arthroscopic classification for basal joint osteoarthritis provides additional clinical information and can direct further treatment depending on the stage of disease. This article reviews the brief history of trapeziometacarpal arthroscopy and provides insight as to how this technique can be added to the surgeon's armamentarium in managing this common condition.

Primary osteoarthritis of the carpometacarpal joint of the thumb is common, especially in women aged 60 or older. Patients usually present with activity-related pain at the thumb base. First treatment may include activity modification, pain relieving medications, splinting, and possibly corticosteroid injections. When these measures fail to preserve or restore the patient's quality of life, surgical intervention may be appropriate. Many surgical alternatives are described for the treatment of thumb carpometacarpal joint arthritis, and most begin with at least partial trapeziectomy. Hematoma-distraction arthroplasty results in improved outcomes as compared with historical results following trapeziectomy alone. Temporary distraction allows the body's healing response to fill in the trapezial void with scar tissue, obviating the need for ligament reconstruction or tissue interposition.

Abductor pollicis longus suspensionplasty is a simple, effective treatment alternative for basal joint arthritis. Use of a suspensionplasty technique acknowledges our current understanding of forces involved during pinch and grip, as well as the role of normal ligamentous anatomy. The primary rationale for performing suspensionplasty revolves around resisting the sagittal plane collapse that will occur when the thumb is loaded during pinch. In the absence of a volar-based suspension of the metacarpal, cantilever bending forces and axial force transmission will result in the dissipation of force along the thumb lever arm, and ultimately longitudinal collapse. Maximal grip and pinch strength require suspensionplasty, which can be performed using a variety of techniques. The author's current technique for suspensionplasty is described.

Silicone implant arthroplasty has been used for more than 40 years for severe rheumatoid disease at the metacarpophalangeal (MCP) joint. Multiple investigations have shown that silicone arthroplasty places the MCP joint in a more extended posture, with some improvement in the total arc of motion. Ulnar drift is also improved, but strength and other objective measures have not demonstrated marked changes postoperatively. The lack of prospective data and more complete outcome assessment has been, at least in part, responsible for the marked difference in opinions between rheumatologists and hand surgeons on the effectiveness of MCP arthroplasty. Recent reports using patient-centered outcome measures have shown that early outcome is favorable, with improvements in appearance, pain, and function.

The metacarpophalangeal (MP) joint allows for a significant portion of hand function. Osteoarthritis, although less prevalent than rheumatoid arthritis, is not uncommon and can render the MP joint nonfunctional. With unconstrained MP joint implants, salvage of this joint may be performed reliably in patients who have primary osteoarthritis and post-traumatic arthritis. Pyrolytic carbon implants offer advantages over previously used implants. Pyrolytic carbon has an elastic modulus similar to cortical bone, which aids in dampening stresses at the bone prosthetic interface and enhances biological fixation. Pyrolytic carbon has also been found to have excellent long-term biological compatibility. This article provides an overview of the indications, technique, and early outcomes for patients undergoing arthroplasty of the MP joint using a pyrolytic carbon implant.

osteoarthritis. Moreover, the thumb is also often diseased, in any where from 68% to 80% of patients who have rheumatoid arthritis. Much attention over the years has been given to the carpalmetacarpal joint of the thumb, whereas the metacarpophalangeal (MP) joint of the thumb remains largely unstudied. The purpose of this article is to review the etiology of thumb MP joint arthritis, and discuss the different treatment options of this condition.

Patients presenting with symptomatic post-traumatic arthritis involving the finger car-pometacarpal (CMC) joints generally complain of localized pain aggravated by gripping, shaking hands, and occupation or sports-specific activities. The majority of these individuals experience episodic, mild symptoms and respond to nonoperative treatment measures. A small percentage require surgical intervention, especially in cases of missed fracture/dislocations and instability. Reconstruction emphasizes stability, with an eye toward mobility for the ulnar column. Degenerative arthritis often manifests as a dorsal bony prominence over the interval between the second and third CMC joints. This osteophytic projection is commonly referred to as a dorsal carpometacarpal boss, and may be surgically excised down to normal articular cartilage if symptoms warrant.

FORTHCOMING ISSUES

RECENT ISSUES

Hand Clin 22 (2006) xi

Preface

Hand Arthritis

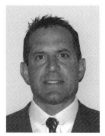

Matthew M. Tomaino, MD, MBA
Guest Editor

Favorable management of the arthritic hand (basal, carpometacarpal, metacarpophalangeal, and interphalangeal joints) in some respects remains invariant—fundamental principles still prevail, arguably, as the most critical aspect of our care. Innovative surgeons continue to refine implant designs, surgical indications, and techniques, however, and this issue of *Hand Clinics* addresses these incremental advances. Students of history will agree that, absent an appreciation thereof, historical blunders may be repeated. And yet, as is often the case, "the more things change, the more they stay the same." In this issue I am grateful for the expert contributions of my colleagues who have been charged with providing enough of a historical backdrop to enable conscientious consideration, and perhaps implementation, of newer developments in the field. Where possible, outcomes have been addressed—a particularly important imperative for each of us in our clinical practices over the next decade—so that we might create value for our patients, exploring new developments when warranted, and relying on time-honored solutions when not.

Matthew M. Tomaino, MD, MBA
University of Rochester Medical Center
601 Elmwood Avenue, Box 665
Rochester, NY 14642, USA

E-mail address:
Matthew_Tomaino@URMC.Rochester.edu

doi:10.1016/j.hcl.2006.02.002

Thumb by Metacarpal Extension Osteotomy: Rationale and Efficacy for Eaton Stage I Disease

Matthew M. Tomaino, MD, MBA

Department of Orthopaedics, Division of Hand, Shoulder and Elbow Surgery,
University of Rochester Medical Center, 601 Elmwood Avenue, Box 665, Rochester, NY 14642, USA

The normal ligamentous anatomy of the thumb basal joint provides extraordinary stability without sacrificing motion [1]. In providing a fixed pivot point at the thumb trapeziometacarpal (TM) joint, substantial cantilever bending forces are resisted, and large loads are accommodated during pinch and grip without subluxation or pain [2,3]. When ligamentous restraint is compromised, however, functional grip and pinch may result in painful synovitis and hypermobility at the TM joint long before the development of cartilage wear and arthritis [4].

This article describes the rationale and results of a "biomechanical" strategy to restore TM stability when symptomatic Eaton Stage I disease exists. Though the author has performed TM arthroscopy, synovectomy, and capsular shrinkage for such cases in 10 patients, I have been dissatisfied with the outcomes, particularly pain relief, and currently rely exclusively on extension osteotomy as treatment for this subset of patients.

Clinical presentation

Radiographs are typically normal, or the TM joint may appear widened, from synovitis. This stage reflects Stage I of the classic Eaton classification of basal joint arthritis. Physical examination may reveal only pain with TM stress and tenderness to palpation beneath the thenar cone (Fig. 1). Deformity, frank instability, subluxation, or crepitance are unusual. It is critical to evaluate the entire hand for signs and symptoms of carpal tunnel syndrome, stenosing flexor tenosynovitis,

DeQuervain's disease, flexor carpi radialis tendonitis, and subsesamoid arthritis. Indeed, when the radiograph is normal and tenderness exists on palpation of the thenar muscles at the level of the TM joint, Stage I disease effectively becomes a diagnosis of exclusion [4,5].

Pathomechanics

Functional incompetence of the basal joint's palmar oblique ligament (POL) results in pathologic laxity, abnormal translation of the metacarpal on the trapezium, and generation of excessive shear forces between the joint surfaces, particularly within the palmar portion of the joint during grip and pinch activity [6,7]. Histologic study has shown that attritional changes in the POL at its attachment to the palmar lip of the metacarpal precede degeneration of cartilage [8].

Cadaveric investigation of acute dislocation of the thumb TM joint has shown that the primary restraint was the dorsoradial (DRL) ligament [9]. Thus the POL and DRL ligament are critical stabilizers of the TM joint during lateral pinch, and when either or both are attenuated or incompetent, some degree of dorsal translation of the metacarpal may cause symptoms of pain. Indeed, though Eaton and Littler [4] recommended ligament reconstruction in 1973 to restore thumb stability in cases of end-stage osteoarthritis, subsequent reports have confirmed its efficacy for early stage disease—the hypermobile TM joint—as well [10,11].

Rationale for osteotomy

Pellegrini and colleagues [12] were the first to evaluate the biomechanical efficacy of extension

E-mail address: matthew_tomaino@urmc.rochester.edu

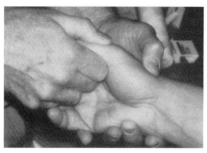

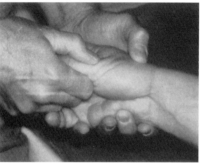

Fig. 1. The trapeziometacarpal stress test.

osteotomy (Fig. 2). Palmar contact area was unloaded with a concomitant shift in contact more dorsally so long as arthrosis did not extend more dorsal than the midpoint of the trapezium. Shrivastava and coworkers [13] studied the effect of a simulated osteotomy on TM joint laxity by flexing the metacarpal base 30°, thus placing the joint in the relationship it would assume if an extension osteotomy was performed (Fig. 3). The

simulated extension osteotomy reduced laxity in all directions tested: dorsal-volar (40% reduction), radial-ulnar (23% reduction), distraction (15% reduction), and pronation-supination (29% reduction). They hypothesized that the beneficial clinical effects of a thumb metacarpal extension osteotomy may be partially caused by tightening of the DRL, which might reduce dorsal translation.

Clinical outcome

In light of Pellegrini's biomechanical data [12] and the author's own relative dissatisfaction with Eaton ligament reconstruction for Stage I disease, primarily related to what seemed to be an 8- to 10-month recovery period and a fairly stiff TM joint, I prospectively evaluated the efficacy of a 30° extension osteotomy in 12 patients (12 thumbs) between 1995 and 1998 [5]. TM arthrotomy allowed accurate intra-articular assessment and verified POL detachment from the metacarpal rim in each case. Follow-up averaged 2.1 years and ranged between 6 and 46 months. All osteotomies healed at an average of 7 weeks. Eleven patients were satisfied with outcome. Grip and pinch strength increased an average of 8.5 and 3 kg, respectively.

Since that study's publication, the author has become even more impressed by the efficacy of the procedure and believe, as Shrivastava and colleagues suggested [13], that osteotomy decreases laxity and shifts contact area more dorsally. It seems logical that the DRL participates in this

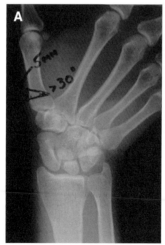
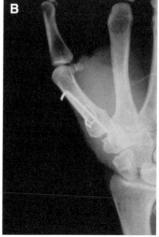

Fig. 2. (*A*) Lateral radiograph shows the anticipated wedge of bone to be resected to afford a 30° extension osteotomy. (*B*) Lateral radiograph after completion of extension osteotomy.

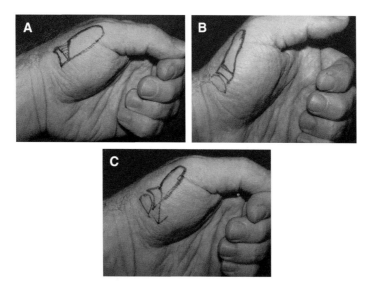

Fig. 3. (*A*) Left thumb in lateral pinch with a planned extension osteotomy diagrammed on the skin. (*B*) Closure of the wedge causes the metacarpal to extend away from the index finger. (*C*) To regain the lateral pinch position, the metacarpal base must flex on the trapezium after extension osteotomy. (*From* Shrivastava N, Koff MF, Abbott AE, et al. Simulated extension osteotomy of the thumb metacarpal reduces carpometacarpal joint laxity in lateral pinch. J Hand Surg [Am] 2003;28:735; with permission.)

effect, and substantiates the contention that the DRL is an important stabilizer [9].

The author's surgical technique has changed little since the publication in 2000, except that I use staples now (OSStaple, Biomedical Enterprises, San Antonio, Texas) to avoid the use of a percutaneously placed Kirschner wire. Further, if I am convinced that the joint surfaces are essentially normal, which I usually assume if the radiograph is normal and there is no crepitance on examination, I do not perform an arthrotomy.

Surgical technique

Regional, axillary block anesthesia is performed and a nonsterile tourniquet is placed. After exsanguination with an Esmarch bandage and inflation of the tourniquet to 250 mmHg, a dorsal incision is made from the base of the thumb metacarpal distally for approximately 3 cm. In the subcutaneous tissue the sensory branches of the radial and lateral antebrachial cutaneous nerves are identified and protected. Subperiosteal exposure is obtained without injuring the extensor pollicis longus, and the TM joint is identified with a 25-gauge needle. One cm distal to the TM joint, near circumferential access around the metacarpal is obtained in anticipation of the osteotomy. The volar extent of the metacarpal is visualized at this location to facilitate accurate resection of

a dorsally based 30° wedge of bone (see Fig. 3). A microsagittal saw is used to score the metacarpal 1 cm distal to its base transversely, but a complete cut through the volar cortex is not made. A new saw blade is left in that partial osteotomy site and a second blade is used approximately 5 mm distal to the first cut at an angle of 30°, so that the two blades intersect at the volar cortex. The wedge of bone is removed, the distal metacarpal is extended and compressed against the proximal fragment, and two 11 × 8 staples are placed (Fig. 4). Typically, the author maintains the reduced position of the metacarpal while my assistant predrills, and then places the staples.

A layered closure of the periosteum and skin is performed, and overlying thumb spica splint is placed for 10 days. After that time sutures are removed and a thumb spica cast with the interphalangeal joint of the thumb left free is placed for an additional 4 weeks. Approximately 6 weeks following surgery, a forearm-based thumb spica orthoplast splint is placed, and the patient is instructed to begin gentle TM motion. Grip and pinch exercises are started at approximately 8 weeks after surgery unless union is delayed.

Discussion

Although the cause of osteoarthritis of the TM joint is probably multifactorial, instability

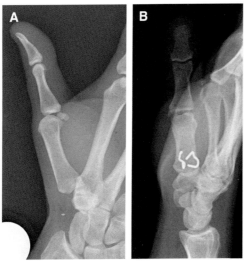

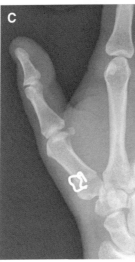

Fig. 4. (*A*) Preoperative lateral radiograph. (*B*) Postoperative posteroanterior radiograph after stabilization with two OSStaple staples. (*C*) Postoperative lateral radiograph after stabilization with two OSStaple staples.

secondary to degeneration of the POL has been implicated. Indeed, the forces experienced at the normal TM joint with grip and pinch are not only magnified severalfold [2,3], but appear to be concentrated in the palmar aspect of the joint. The observation that ligament reconstruction of the painful TM joint is successful treatment for Eaton Stage I disease reflects the importance of the POL and DRL in providing stability to the joint [7,9] and in limiting dorsal translation of the metacarpal, which normally occurs with dynamic pinch activity.

The precise role of thumb metacarpal extension osteotomy for the hypermobile TM joint is no longer ill-defined. Biomechanical and clinical data validate the rationale and favorable outcome. The precise mechanism for pain relief is not known, but it is probably a combination of load transfer and diminished laxity. Because extension osteotomy shifts mechanical loading at the TM joint more dorsally and redirects force vectors, fixed subluxation or multidirectional instability contraindicate the procedure. Indeed, a preoperative TM stress test is meant to provoke pain related to POL incompetence only. More global instability may reflect a greater degree of capsuloligamentous injury, and may necessitate ligament reconstruction [4].

In summary, pre- and postoperative subjective and objective assessment has allowed a comprehensive analysis of outcome following a 30° extension osteotomy of the thumb metacarpal [5]. Excellent pain relief and improved grip and pinch strength compare favorably with those published following ligament reconstruction [10,11]. For Eaton Stage I disease of the TM joint, this procedure appears to be an efficacious alternative to ligament reconstruction. Further, it has been the author's personal observation that this procedure provides more reliable pain relief than TM arthroscopy, synovectomy, and capsular shrinkage.

References

[1] Bettinger P, Lindschied Berger R, et al. An anatomic study of the stabilizing ligaments of the trapezium and trapeziometacarpal joint. J Hand Surg [Am] 1999;24:786–98.

[2] Cooney W, Chao E. Biomechanical analysis of static forces in the thumb during hand function. J Bone Joint Surg [Am] 1977;59:27.

[3] Imaeda T, Niebur G, Cooney WP III, et al. Kinematics of the normal trapeziometacarpal joint. J Orthop Res 1994;12:197–204.

[4] Eaton RG, Littler JW Jr. Ligament reconstruction of the painful thumb carpometacarpal joint. J Bone Joint Surg [Am] 1973;55:1655–66.

[5] Tomaino MM. Treatment of Eaton Stage I trapeziometacarpal disease with thumb metacarpal extension osteotomy. J Hand Surg [Am] 2000;25:1100–6.

[6] Pellegrini VD. Osteoarthritis of the thumb trapeziometacarpal joint: a study of the pathophysiology of articular cartilage degeneration. II. Articular wear patterns in the osteoarthritic joint. J Hand Surg [Am] 1991;16:975–82.

[7] Pellegrini VD, Olcott CW, Hollenberg G. Contact patterns in the trapeziometacarpal joint: the role of the palmar beak ligament. J Hand Surg [Am] 1993; 18:238–44.

[8] Doerschuk SH, Hicks DG, Chinchilli VM, et al. Histopathology of the palmar beak ligament in trapeziometacarpal osteoarthritis. J Hand Surg [Am] 1999;24:496–504.

[9] Strauch RJ, Behrman MJ, Rosenwasser MP. A biomechanical assessment of ligaments preventing dorsoradial subluxation of the trapeziometacarpal joint. J Hand Surg [Am] 1998;23:607–11.

[10] Eaton RG, Lane LB, Littler JW, et al. Ligament reconstruction for the painful thumb carpometacarpal joint: a long-term assessment. J Hand Surg [Am] 1984;9:692–9.

[11] Freedman DM, Eaton RG, Glickel SZ. Long-term results of volarv ligament reconstruction for symptomatic basal joint laxity. J Hand Surg [Am] 2000; 25:297–304.

[12] Pellegrini VD, Parentis M, Judkins A, et al. Extension metacarpal osteotomy in the treatment of trapeziometacarpal osteoarthritis: A biomechanical study. J Hand Surg [Am] 1996;21:16–23.

[13] Shrivastava N, Koff MF, Abbot AE, et al. Simulated extension osteotomy of the thumb metacarpal reduces carpometacarpal joint laxity in lateral pinch. J Hand Surg [Am] 2003;28:733–8.

ELSEVIER
SAUNDERS

Hand Clin 22 (2006) 143–151

HAND
CLINICS

Ligament Reconstruction

Steven Z. Glickel, MD[a,b,]*, Salil Gupta, MD[b]

[a]*Department of Orthopedic Surgery, Columbia University College of Physicians and Surgeons, 622 West 168 Street,*
New York, NY 10032, USA
[b]*C.V. Starr Hand Surgery Center, St. Luke's-Roosevelt Hospital Center, 1000 Tenth Avenue,*
New York, NY 10019, USA

Eaton and Littler [1] described the staging system for basal joint disease that has remained most widely used for the past 30 years. That staging system is based upon the true lateral radiograph of the thumb and defines the degree of involvement of the carpometacarpal (CMC) and scaphotrapezial (ST) joints. In Stage I disease, the articular contours are normal. There is occasional joint space widening caused by effusion or ligament laxity. Stage I disease, therefore, is "prearthritic." Stage II disease has mild joint space narrowing, minimal subchondral sclerosis, and joint debris or osteophytes measuring 2 mm or less in diameter. The intraoperative findings in Stage II disease vary from mild fibrillation and thinning of the articular cartilage to advanced disease with areas of eburnation. Volar ligament reconstruction is indicated for the treatment of Stage I or early Stage II disease, in which the changes in the articular cartilage are mild. The rationale for volar ligament reconstruction is to stabilize the CMC joint and reduce the shear forces that cause the synovitis of Stage I disease and the progression of the articular changes in Stage II disease.

The literature concerning stabilization of the lax thumb CMC joint is quite limited. Slocum [2] described stabilizing the joint for CMC dislocation using a free tendon graft placed through drill holes in the trapezium and thumb metacarpal base. He reported good results in one patient. Bunnell [3] described unsatisfactory results using this technique. Cho [4] stabilized a chronically subluxated thumb CMC joint with a distally based strip of the abductor pollicis longus (APL) tendon secured to the trapezium. The patient treated with this technique had full pain-free range of motion 18 months after the procedure. Eggers [5] mobilized a radial strip of the extensor carpi radialis longus (ECRL) tendon, leaving it attached distally. He placed it through two holes in the thumb metacarpal base to stabilize the CMC joint. Kestler [6] reported a case in which the CMC joint was stabilized using a distally based strip of the extensor pollicis brevis (EPB) tendon placed from distal to proximal through gouge holes in the dorsum of the thumb metacarpal and trapezium respectively. The tendon was sutured back to itself. Although he reported a satisfactory result in one male patient treated with this procedure, he concluded that a more physiologic reconstruction would be to use a strip of APL tendon left attached distally and placed through two gouge holes in the dorsum of the trapezium, looped back on itself, and sutured [6].

Eaton and Littler published a paper entitled "Ligament Reconstruction for the Painful Thumb Carpometacarpal Joint" in 1973 [1]. They described a surgical technique for stabilization of the thumb CMC joint that became commonly known as "volar ligament reconstruction." In that same paper, they proposed a staging system for osteoarthritis of the basal joint of the thumb, which they and others subsequently revised to its current form in a later, long-term follow-up study [7]. The surgical technique involved mobilizing approximately 50% of the width of the flexor carpi radialis (FCR) tendon from proximal to distal, leaving it attached to the index metacarpal. A gouge hole was made from dorsal to volar in the base of the index metacarpal. The tendon strip

---

* Corresponding Author. C.V. Starr Hand Surgery Center, St. Luke's-Roosevelt Hospital Center, 1000 Tenth Avenue, New York, NY 10019.

E-mail address: sglickel@MSN.com (S.Z. Glickel).

was passed from volar to dorsal through that gouge hole, and then from dorsal to volar looping it around the intact FCR, to which it was sutured. In that seminal article, the volar ligament reconstruction was used in patients who had all four stages of basal joint disease. The researchers achieved excellent results in five patients who had Stage I or II disease [1]. The results were not as good in Stage III and IV disease. In their medium-term follow-up study in 1984 on a larger series of patients [7], good or excellent results were achieved in 95% of 20 patients who had Stage I or II disease.

The study authors recognized that the procedure is primarily indicated for those patients who have symptomatic laxity of the basal joint without established degenerative disease. The procedure used today is not significantly different from that originally described by Eaton and Littler in 1973 [1]. The only real modification has been to harvest the strip of FCR tendon subcutaneously beneath one long skin bridge instead of mobilizing the tendon beneath multiple skin bridges created by short, transverse incisions on the volar aspect of the forearm.

Indications

Laxity of the CMC joint of the thumb may be a manifestation of generalized ligament laxity, result as the sequela of trauma, or be a manifestation of metabolic disease such as Ehlers-Danlos syndrome. It is seen most commonly as one manifestation of generalized ligament laxity, particularly in young women in the third to fourth decades of life. They typically also have hyperextension of the elbows, knees, and finger metacarpophalangeal (MP) joints. The symptoms are exacerbated by activity, but are not caused by trauma. A much smaller subset of patients have basal joint laxity resulting from trauma. Dislocations of the CMC joint are uncommon, but cause laxity both acutely and chronically. Irreducible dislocations, or those that remain unstable after reduction, are candidates for volar ligament reconstruction. Simorian and Trumble [8] have recommended volar ligament reconstruction for all patients who have CMC dislocations, citing improved long-term results compared with reduction without reconstruction. Rare patients have chronic pain resulting from Grade III sprains of the ligaments of the CMC joint.

Patients who have symptomatic basal joint laxity typically present with pain in the thenar eminence. They generally do not localize the pain to the area of the CMC joint, and might characterize it as radiating distally. The pain tends to be exacerbated by forceful pinch, as in writing, or by activities requiring torsional motions with the involved hand, such as unscrewing jar tops or turning doorknobs. Holding large objects requiring maximal abduction of the thumb while flexing against resistance, as in holding a half-gallon container of milk, may be painful as well. The pain is typically aching in character. As the symptoms become more severe, the pain may be present at rest as well as with activity. Clinical signs of symptomatic laxity of the thumb CMC joint include tenderness, particularly of the radiovolar aspect of the joint, and hypermobility when the joint is stressed radially and dorsally. In patients who have Stage I subluxation, there is no crepitus with CMC range of motion, because the articular cartilage is intact. Patients who have Stage II disease may have mild crepitus with passive manipulation of the joint. Axial compression with rotation of the CMC joint (grind test) is often minimally painful or not painful. Axial traction with rotation of the joint (distraction test) may be painful because of traction on an inflamed joint capsule. The shear test is often negative because the articular surfaces are intact [9].

Radiographic assessment Includes standard posteranterior (PA), lateral, and oblique views of the thumb. The lateral radiograph should be a true lateral, in which the sesamoids of the thumb MP joint overlap each other. This is the view used for staging the disease. In addition, a stress view of the basal joint as described by Eaton and Littler [1] may be useful to demonstrate laxity of the CMC joint. The stress view is a PA view of the basal joint of the thumb shot while the patient pushes the lateral aspect of both thumb tips against each other. This tends to force the thumb metacarpal base radially, subluxating it out of the trapezial saddle.

Conservative treatment of Stage I disease includes immobilization of the joint with a long opponens thermoplastic splint, immobilizing the wrist, thumb CMC, and thumb MP joints [10]. The efficacy of splinting has been confirmed by Swigart and colleagues [10] and Weiss and coworkers [11]. Alternatively, the joint may be adequately immobilized, particularly during work activities, with a short opponens splint that does not fully immobilize wrist, but stabilizes the basal joint [11]. This may be combined with nonsteroidal anti-inflammatory medication.

Immobilization should continue for a period of at least 1 month, after which the patient should be reassessed. If the symptoms are improving but not completely resolved, the period of immobilization can be extended. If the symptoms do not improve or plateau, the pain may be improved by injection of the CMC joint with corticosteroid. The number of injections should be limited to prevent damage to the articular cartilage. The authors' preference is to limit the number of injections to two. The majority of patients do improve with this treatment regimen. Patients who fail conservative treatment are candidates for volar ligament reconstruction.

The rationale for volar ligament reconstruction is that the symptoms arise from synovitis caused by shear forces on the CMC joint. The shear forces result from ligament laxity, which allows translation of the metacarpal on the trapezium with axial and torsional loading [1]. Ligament reconstruction stabilizes the joint and reduces those shear forces. There and is some disagreement in the literature as to which ligament is most responsible for stabilizing the CMC joint and which ligament is reconstructed by the technique described herein. Several authors, including Eaton and Littler [1], Pellegrini [12], and Tomaino and colleagues [13], believe that the volar (anterior oblique or beak) ligament is the principal stabilizer of the thumb CMC joint. Others, including Strauch and colleagues [14], feel that the dorsoradial ligament is the primary stabilizer, particularly in providing the restraint to dorsal dislocation. The technique of volar ligament reconstruction makes this argument somewhat moot, because the manner in which the FCR tendon slip is routed functionally reconstructs both the anterior oblique and dorsoradial ligaments.

Surgical technique

The basal joint of the thumb is exposed through a modified Wagner incision. There is a longitudinal component parallel to the long axis of the thumb metacarpal located in the interval between the glabrous palmar and nonglabrous dorsal skin. The incision is continued transversely in the wrist crease to just ulnar to the FCR tendon (Fig. 1). There is invariably a branch of the dorsal sensory branch of the radial nerve crossing the operative field that should be mobilized and protected throughout the procedure.

The radial edge of the thenar musculature at its insertion on the thumb metacarpal is identified

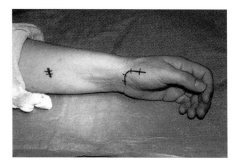

Fig. 1. The basal joint is exposed through a modified Wagner incision, with the longitudinal limb in the interval between the palmar glabrous and dorsal nonglabrous skin. The proximal incision is for harvest of the FCR tendon.

and the muscle elevated extraperiosteally from the thumb metacarpal, thus exposing the metacarpal base, CMC joint, and trapezium. Most patients undergoing volar ligament reconstruction have normal-appearing CMC joints on radiograph and are symptomatically lax. There is usually no crepitus with motion of the CMC joint. In that situation, it is unnecessary to visualize the CMC joint. If, however, there is any question about the condition of the articular cartilage, a transverse arthrotomy can be made and the joint inspected. The arthrotomy should be closed after exploration.

The skin flaps are elevated sufficiently far dorsally to visualize the dorsum of the metacarpal base. The interval between the extensor pollicis longus (EPL) and EPB tendons is developed, and the dorsal cortex exposed. A hole is made in the base of the thumb metacarpal from dorsal to volar, parallel and approximately 1.0 cm distal to the articular surface. The hole is begun in a plane perpendicular to the axis of the thumbnail, and is made with handheld gouges (Fig. 2). There are three sizes of gouge with progressively larger radii of curvature of the cutting end. The small gouge is carefully driven through the metacarpal base to emerge volarly just distal to the normal insertion of the volar (anterior oblique) ligament. The hole is enlarged with the medium and large gouges sequentially. A 28-gauge stainless steel wire is placed through the hole from volar to dorsal, using the concavity of the gouge as a guide for passage (Fig. 3). The two ends of the wire are clamped in a hemostat.

Attention is then directed to harvesting a slip of the FCR tendon. The sheath of the FCR tendon is identified in the transverse limb of the surgical incision at the level of the wrist crease.

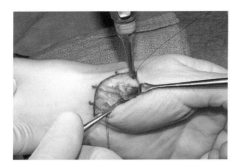

Fig. 2. A hole is made in the base of the thumb metacarpal with a handheld gouge. The hole is approximately 1 cm distal to the articular surface. A 28-gauge stainless steel wire is placed through the hole for later passage of the FCR tendon.

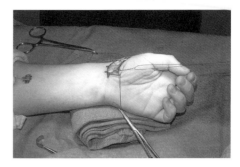

Fig. 4. One half of the FCR is harvested through a 2-cm incision in the forearm over the musculotendinous junction. A braided 28-gauge wire is passed from proximal to distal along the FCR to draw an 0-prolene suture from distal to proximal to be used to split the FCR longitudinally.

The tendon sheath is opened proximally and distally for approximately 1 cm in each direction. The traditional way to harvest the FCR tendon is through multiple short transverse incisions on the volar forearm, between the incision at the wrist and the level of the musculotendinous junction of the tendon. After it is mobilized proximally, the slip of the FCR tendon is dissected and passed from proximal to distal beneath the skin bridges between the incisions.

It is possible to harvest the slip of FCR through the transverse limb of the incision at the wrist crease and only one incision in the forearm at the musculotendinous junction (Fig. 4). To accomplish this, the plane between the subcutaneous tissue and the FCR tendon sheath is developed. The tendon sheath is incised longitudinally under direct vision proximally and distally. The tendon is mobilized at the musculotendinous junction and delivered into the wound. The tendon is split longitudinally in approximately the midline. The fibers of the FCR spiral, so the fibers that begin

ulnarly terminate radially, and it is this part of the tendon that should be mobilized. Therefore, the ulnar half of the tendon is transected and dissected distally for a few centimeters. The tendon is split longitudinally with a heavy suture placed into the split between the halves of the tendon. To deliver that suture into the forearm wound, the suture must be drawn from the distal incision proximally. A 28-gauge stainless steel wire is bent in half. The apex of the bend is placed into a skin hook and the wire twisted, leaving a small loop on the end. This wire is semirigid, which facilitates its passage. It is placed in the forearm wound and carefully threaded in the subfascial plane toward the wrist along the course of the FCR tendon (Fig. 5). The looped end of the wire is passed into the transverse limb of the Wagner incision, and a 0-prolene suture is placed through the loop and folded onto itself. The two ends of the suture are held in a hemostat at the wrist, and the folded end is drawn into the forearm incision.

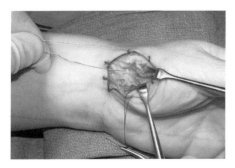

Fig. 3. The wire will be used to draw the FCR tendon slip from volar to dorsal through the hole in the metacarpal base.

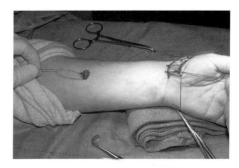

Fig. 5. The 0-prolene suture is brought into the forearm wound and the braided wire loop is removed from the suture.

The loop of the wire is cut and the wire removed. The folded prolene suture is then placed in the crotch of the split FCR tendon (Fig. 6). The divided end of the tendon is held with the hemostat and the suture is pulled from proximal to distal into the wrist incision, splitting the tendon along its fibers (Fig. 7).

The split in the tendon is further developed distal to the level of the bercle of the trapezium. The end of the FCR tendon slip is secured in a knotted loop of the volar end of the stainless steel wire, previously placed in the hole in the metacarpal base. Using the wire for traction, the tendon graft is delivered through the hole from volar to dorsal. The thumb is reduced in a position of extension and abduction. Tension is set on the tendon by pulling it firmly, and then allowing it to retract 2 or 3 mm as the tension is relaxed. The FCR segment is sutured to the periosteum adjacent to the hole in the dorsal cortex of the metacarpal, using figure-of-eight or mattress sutures of 3-0 braided synthetic suture such as ethibond (Fig. 8). The tendon is placed beneath the APL tendon to which it is sutured (Fig. 9). It is directed volarly, where it is looped around the intact FCR tendon, to which it is also sutured (Fig. 10). Any remaining length of tendon is redirected dorsally, where it is passed beneath and sutured to the abductor pollicis longus tendon.

The stability of the CMC joint should be assessed before closure. The reconstruction is secure, and it is not necessary to transfix the CMC joint with a Kirschner wire, although there is little harm in doing so if it provides the operator an additional sense of security. The thenar musculature is reapproximated with interrupted sutures of 4-0 PDS or vicryl. The skin is closed with

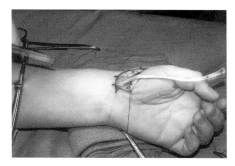

Fig. 7. The split FCR is delivered into the distal wound.

interrupted sutures of 5-0 plain or vicryl rapide, which obviates the need for a cast change to remove sutures. The thumb is immobilized in a short arm-thumb spica cast for a period of 4 weeks, after which it may be immobilized part time in a thumb stabilizer splint, which is removed for range-of-motion exercise.

Several key steps of the procedure are shown in illustrations done by one of the creators of the procedure, Dr. J. William Littler (Figs. 11 and 12) [15].

Therapy

The postoperative cast remains on for 1 month. When the cast is removed, the patient is referred to the hand therapist, who provides a customized, thermoplastic, long opponens splint. The splint is worn for protection and removed for exercise. The patient works on active and active-assisted range of motion of the wrist and thumb CMC, MP, and interphalangeal (IP) joints. Palmar abduction of the thumb is begun first, followed by radial abduction. The patient is instructed to move from a position of palmar abduction to radial abduction

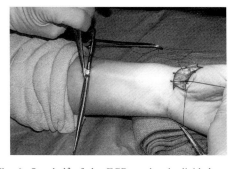

Fig. 6. One half of the FCR tendon is divided proximally and the 0-prolene suture is used to split the tendon longitudinally by pulling it firmly from proximal to distal.

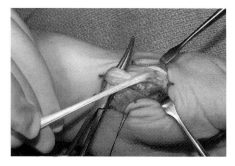

Fig. 8. The FCR tendon slip is drawn through the hole in the thumb metacarpal base from volar to dorsal using the previously placed wire. The tension is set on the reconstruction and the FCR is sutured to the adjacent periosteum with a 3-0 braided synthetic suture.

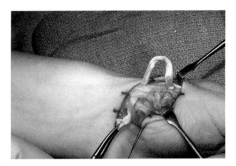

Fig. 9. The FCR tendon slip is passed deep to the APL tendon to which it is sutured.

and then relax. Opposition of the thumb to the index and long fingers is encouraged during the first 2 weeks out of plaster, avoiding opposition to the ring and small fingers so as to not stress the reconstructed ligament. Patients massage the scar several times per day. Gentle tip-to-tip pinch is begun to work on dexterity.

Opposition to the ring and small fingers is begun 2 weeks after cast removal. At this point, thumb flexion is increased by flexing from the tip to the base of the index and long fingers, followed by flexion along the ring and small fingers to the base during the next 2 weeks. During this same period, 2 weeks after cast removal, the patient exercises to maximize abduction.

Strengthening is initiated 1 month after cast removal. Tip-to-tip, key pinch, and grip strengthening are begun with minimal resistance putty and progressively increased. Patients are allowed essentially unrestricted activity 3 months postoperatively.

Results

There are a limited number of studies in the literature reporting results of volar ligament

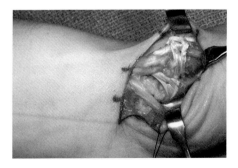

Fig. 10. The FCR slip is then passed around the intact FCR tendon volarly and then back dorsally, where it is sutured to itself.

reconstruction of the thumb CMC joint. These studies do, however, demonstrate consistently excellent or good results in patients who have Stage I or II disease.

In 1973 Eaton and Littler [1], in their seminal paper describing the technique of volar ligament reconstruction for the painful thumb CMC joint, reported results in 18 patients who were followed for an average of 30.9 months. Two patients had Stage I disease, 3 had Stage II, 8 had Stage III, and 5 had Stage IV disease. Eleven of 18 patients had excellent results, 5 were good, and 2 were fair. There were no failures. Symptoms in all patients improved postoperatively. When only patients who had Stage I and II disease were considered, results were uniformly excellent. The patient grading at the 12 months postoperatively remained the same for the duration of the follow-up. The authors concluded that results were proportional to the degree of articular damage. Patients who had minimal articular deterioration (Stage I or II) had excellent results. The authors recommended alternative treatments for those who have deterioration beyond Stage III disease [1].

In 1984 Eaton and colleagues [7] reviewed the results of their first fifty volar ligament reconstructions. Thirty-eight reconstructions were available for follow-up at an average of 7.1 years. With all stages of disease considered collectively, there were good or excellent results in 84% and fair results in 16%. All 8 Stage I thumbs had excellent results, and 91% of Stage II thumbs had good or excellent results. With Stage I and Stage II cases combined, 18 of 19, or 95%, had good or excellent results. Pain was eliminated or dramatically improved in all patients. Seventeen of 19 patients who had Stage I or II disease were pain-free. All thumbs were stable, except one in which the instability was mild. Pinch strength was 90% or more than the contralateral thumb in 34 of 38 thumbs. The authors assessed extension-abduction by the ability to flatten the palm on a countertop, and flexion-adduction by the ability to oppose the tip of the thumb to the head of the fifth metacarpal. Extension-abduction was slightly reduced in 53%, and normal flexion-adduction was achieved in 95%. At final follow-up, none of the Stage I thumbs progressed to a more advanced stage of disease. Ninety percent of the Stage II cases remained Stage II. The 2 Stage II patients who progressed were noted to have significant cartilage attrition when the joint was inspected at surgery. Twenty percent of the Stage III cases went on to Stage IV. Two of the

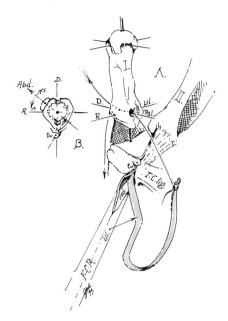

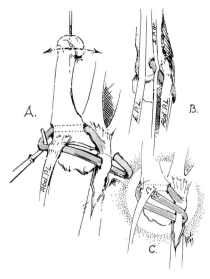

Fig. 11. (*A*) View from the volar aspect of the wrist and thumb. The FCR tendon slip has been mobilized and its proximal end secured with the previously placed stainless steel wire. The gouge hole is shown in the volar midline of the thumb metacarpal base, through which the tendon is drawn from volar to dorsal. (*B*) Axial view of the thumb metacarpal base shows the relationship of the dorsal gouge hole to the APL tendon. The hole is placed just ulnar to the midline of the thumb metacarpal base. The normal volar ligament inserts just ulnar to the midline of the thumb metacarpal base. The ligament reconstruction does not correspond exactly to the obliquity of the normal ligament from the trapezial tubercle (tu) to its insertion, but does provide a strong mechanical restraint. Abd, abduction; D, dorsal; p, pronation; Pal, palmar; R, radial; S, supination; T.C. lig, transverse carpal ligament; Ul, ulnar. (*From* Glickel SZ. Stabilization of CMC joint. In: Strickland JW, editor. The hand. 1st edition. Philadelphia: Lippincott-Raven Publishers; 1998. p. 387; with permission.)

9 Stage IV cases eventually required trapeziectomy and implant arthroplasty, and one fused spontaneously. The authors concluded that "ligament reconstruction is recommended only for patients in Stage I and Stage II disease" [7].

Lane and Eaton [16] reported the results of 42 volar ligament reconstructions, with an average follow-up interval of 5.2 years for 25 thumbs that had Stage I disease and 4.8 years for 17 that had Stage II. The results were excellent or good in all cases of Stage I disease and in 82% of Stage II disease. Eighteen percent of Stage II cases had fair results. Seventy-two percent of

Fig. 12. (*A*) The FCR tendon slip (*shaded*) has been placed through the volar/dorsal gouge hole in the thumb metacarpal base and beneath the abductor pollicis longus tendon. A probe is beneath the tendon dorsally. The tendon is directed volarly along the radial side of the carpometacarpal joint and is passed beneath the intact FCR tendon. (*B*) Dorsal view of the operative field showing the emergence of the FCR tendon slip (*shaded*) through the dorsal gouge hole. The tendon exits the bone beneath the extensor pollicis brevis and is placed deep to the APL tendon on the dorsoradial side of the metacarpal base. (*C*) The reconstruction is completed by passing the FCR tendon slip beneath the intact part of the FCR volarly and then back dorsally beneath the APL tendon to which it is sutured. Abd.P.L., abduction pollicis longus; E.P.L., extensor pollicis longus. (*From* Glickel SZ. Stabilization of CMC joint. In: Strickland JW, editor. The hand. 1st edition. Philadelphia: Lippincott-Raven Publishers; 1998. p. 388; with permission.)

Stage I cases had complete pain relief; the remaining 28% had mild pain with strenuous use. Of the Stage II cases, 70% reported complete or minimal pain and 30% reported mild to moderate pain with average use. All patients had less pain than preoperatively. Pinch strength was 90% or greater than the contralateral side in 92% of the Stage I cases and in 88% of the Stage II cases. All patients retained their flexion-adduction motion, and 50% of all cases had a decrease in the "palm flat test." The authors believed the inability to flatten the palm represented "tightness" of the ligament reconstruction. There was no correlation between the results of the palm flat test and the ultimate result. None of the 21 Stage I cases had radiographic progression of disease at final follow-up.

Three cases, 18%, of Stage II disease progressed to Stage III disease. Each of these cases was noted to have had significant cartilage degeneration intraoperatively interphalangeal (IP) [16].

Freedman and coworkers [17] reported long-term results of ligament reconstruction, with a minimum of 10-year follow-up in 24 thumbs in 19 patients who had Stage I or II disease. The mean follow-up was 15 years. Twenty-three thumbs were Stage I. Seven thumbs were pain-free, 13 had pain with strenuous activity, and 4 had pain with activities of daily living. All patients reported improvement in pain postoperatively. Radial and palmar abduction of the affected thumb and pinch strength were not significantly different from the contralateral side. Eighty-seven percent of the thumbs were stable to stress testing; 13% had some residual laxity. The authors suggest that volar ligament reconstruction may slow or prevent progression of articular degeneration of the CMC joint. At final follow-up, 15 thumbs were categorized as Stage I disease, 7 as Stage II, and 2 as Stage III disease. Hence, 15 thumbs did not progress to a higher stage, 6 thumbs advanced one stage, and 2 thumbs advanced two stages [17]. Only two thumbs (8%) at final follow-up had Stage III or IV disease, compared with prevalence rates of 17% to 33% reported for the normal population [18,19], suggesting that the procedure may slow disease progression.

In 2001, Lane and Henly [20] reported the results of 37 consecutive volar ligament reconstructions in 35 patients who had Stage I disease followed for an average 5.2 years. Sixty-seven percent of thumbs had excellent, 30% had good results, and 3% had poor results. Sixty-seven percent had complete resolution of preoperative pain, and 30% were markedly improved. One poor result was salvaged with arthrodesis. All thumbs were stable to stress at final follow-up, and all patients returned to work or sports postoperatively. At final follow-up, none of the thumbs, including 7 followed for 10 years or more, had radiographic evidence of arthritic degeneration [20].

Summary

Volar ligament reconstruction is an effective technique for treating symptomatic laxity of the CMC joint of the thumb. The laxity may be a manifestation of generalized ligament laxity, post-traumatic, or metabolic (Ehler-Danlos). The reconstruction reduces the shear forces on the joint that contribute to the development and persistence of inflammation. Although there have been only a few reports of the results of volar ligament reconstruction, the use of the procedure to treat Stage I and Stage II disease gives good to excellent results consistently. More advanced stages of disease are best treated by trapeziectomy, with or without ligament reconstruction.

References

[1] Eaton RG, Littler JW. Ligament reconstruction for the painful thumb carpometacarpal joint. J Bone Joint Surg Am 1973;55A(8):1655–66.

[2] Slocum DB. Stabilization of the articulation of the greater multiangular and the first metacarpal. J Bone Joint Surg 1943;25:626–30.

[3] Bunnell S. Surgery of the hand. 3rd edition. Philadelphia: Lippincott; 1956. p. 345–8.

[4] Cho RO. Translocation of abductor pollicis longus tendon: a treatment for chronic subluxation of the thumb carpometacarpal joint. J Bone Joint Surg 1970;52A:1166–70.

[5] Eggers GWN. Chronic dislocation of the base of the metacarpal of the thumb. J Bone Joint Surg 1945;27: 500–1.

[6] Kestler OC. Recurrent dislocation of the first carpometacarpal joint repaired by functional tenodesis. J Bone Joint Surg 1946;28:858–61.

[7] Eaton RG, Lane LB, Littler JW, et al. Ligament reconstruction for the painful thumb carpometacarpal joint: a long-term assessment. J Hand Surg [Am] 1984;9(5):692–9.

[8] Simonian PT, Trumble TE. Traumatic dislocation of the thumb carpometacarpal joint: early ligamentous reconstruction versus closed reduction and pinning. J Hand Surg [Am] 1996;21(5):802–6.

[9] Eaton RG, Glickel SZ. Trapeziometacarpal osteoarthritis. Staging as a rationale for treatment. Hand Clin 1987;3(4):455–71.

[10] Swigart CR, Eaton RG, Glickel SZ, et al. Splinting in the treatment of arthritis of the first carpometacarpal joint. J Hand Surg [Am] 1999;24(1):86–91.

[11] Weiss S, LaStayo P, Mills A, et al. Prospective analysis of splinting the first carpometacarpal joint: an objective, subjective, and radiographic assessment. J Hand Ther 2000;13(3):218–26.

[12] Pellegrini VD Jr. Osteoarthritis of the trapeziometacarpal joint: the pathophysiology of articular cartilage degeneration. I. Anatomy and pathology of the aging joint. J Hand Surg [Am] 1991;16(6): 967–74.

[13] Tomaino MM, Pellegrini VD Jr, Burton RI. Arthroplasty of the basal joint of the thumb. Long-term follow-up after ligament reconstruction with tendon interposition. J Bone Joint Surg Am 1995;77(3): 346–55.

[14] Strauch RJ, Rosenwasser MP, Behrman MJ. A biomechanical assessment of ligaments preventing dorsoradial subluxation of the trapeziometacarpal joint. J Hand Surg [Am] 1999;24(1):198–9.

[15] Glickel SZ. Stabilization of CMC Joint. In: Strickland JW, editor. The hand. 1st edition. Philadelphia: Lippincott-Raven Publishers; 1998. p. 388–91.

[16] Lane LB, Eaton RG. Ligament reconstruction for the painful "prearthritic" thumb carpometacarpal joint. Clin Orthop Relat Res 1987;220:52–7.

[17] Freedman DM, Eaton RG, Glickel SZ. Long-term results of volar ligament reconstruction for symptomatic basal joint laxity. J Hand Surg [Am] 2000;25(2):297–304.

[18] Armstrong AL, Hunter JB, Davis TR. The prevalence of degenerative arthritis of the base of the thumb in post-menopausal women. J Hand Surg [Br] 1994;19(3):340–1.

[19] Kellgren JH, Lawrence JS. Osteo-arthrosis and disk degeneration in an urban population. Ann Rheum Dis 1958;17(4):388–97.

[20] Lane LB, Henley DH. Ligament reconstruction of the painful, unstable, nonarthritic thumb carpometacarpal joint. J Hand Surg [Am] 2001;26(4):686–91.

Trapeziometacarpal Arthroscopy: A Classification and Treatment Algorithm

Alejandro Badia, MD, FACS[a,b,*]

[a]Miami Hand Center, 8905 SW 87th Avenue, Miami, FL 33176, USA
[b]Department of Small Joint Arthroscopy, DaVinci Learning Center, Miami, FL, USA

Osteoarthritis of the thumb trapeziometacarpal joint is a common clinical problem as well as a perplexing challenge, because of a myriad of treatment options. The fact that so many different surgical options exist for this condition attests to the fact that none of them has an optimal success rate. Or perhaps it may be that the majority of treatment options work to the satisfaction of the surgeon; hence the clinician continues to use his favorite technique, despite the fact that it may not be the most appropriate method for a particular stage of disease. One thing is indisputable: basal joint osteoarthritis of the thumb has many different clinical presentations, and one technique cannot be used for all of the different stages and all patients' individual needs. When conservative treatment has been exhausted, there are a wide range of surgical options to choose from. Treatment should be tailored to the individual patient.

The early stages of basal joint osteoarthritis are most commonly seen in middle-aged women. The literature discusses this in many instances, but rarely gives a solution to the management of these frequently active patients. The use of anti-inflammatories, splinting, and corticosteroid injections serve only as palliative measures, with none of them altering joint mechanics or affecting the articular surface itself in any manner. Moreover, the use of injectable steroids can accelerate cartilage loss and worsen capsular attenuation. Only the mildest cases of transient synovitis will escape the inevitable progressive loss of cartilage,

and hence the need for surgical treatment if the patient indeed wants a definitive solution. After the relatively unimportant distal interphalangeal joint, the thumb carpometacarpal (CMC) joint remains the most common location for osteoarthritis in the hand. It is also the most critical for hand function. The argument has been made that man's evolution has been largely due to the increased range of motion and function as a consequence of the thumb basal joint, which has led to the progressive use of tools in hominid evolution. Treatment of this functionally important joint remains a priority for the hand surgeon, and it is important to use the wide variety of surgical techniques to optimally manage this condition.

Classically, the basal joint has been treated by surgical means only when conservative options have been exhausted. The principal option has been, and remains, some type of open resectional arthroplasty. Although the literature demonstrates good results in many different studies and using a variety of techniques, it remains clear that this is a surgically aggressive procedure, because resection of an entire carpal bone is required to achieve pain relief. This certainly makes good sense in the most advanced cases in which the trapezium is typically flattened or has severe deformity including marginal osteophytes, but earlier stages demand a more conservative option that allows for future interventions if the primary treatment is not successful. Other options, perhaps less aggressive, include arthrodesis, which can provide excellent pain relief but has the obvious limitation of loss of motion, or joint replacement. Joint arthroplasty, as in any other joint in the body, has the added risk of failure of the implant, whether it be silicone or of metallic and plastic components. This is not

* Miami Hand Center, 8905 SW 87th Avenue, Miami, FL 33176.
E-mail address: info@drbadia.com

a good option for the younger, high-demand patients.

History

The advent of small-joint arthroscopic technology has allowed us to apply the concept of minimally invasive surgery to smaller joints, including the wrist, ankle, and now the smaller joints of the hand. Yung-Cheng Chen's classic paper in 1979 [1] on arthroscopy of the wrist and finger joints discussed the feasibility of performing small-joint arthroscopic procedures using the Watanabe No. 24 arthroscope as early as 1970; however, within that paper there was no mention of arthroscopy of the thumb trapeziometacarpal joint, despite the fact that this may be the arthroscope's greatest application. In Chen's paper there was a detailed description of arthroscopy of the wrist, metacarpophalangeal joints, and even the small interphalangeal joints. Nevertheless, the common applicability of this technology to such a ubiquitous clinical scenario may be its greatest contribution [1].

The first clinical paper in the literature on basal joint arthroscopy was written by J. Menon in the *Journal of Arthroscopic and Related Surgery* in 1996 [2]. This paper, "Arthroscopic Management of Trapeziometacarpal Joint Arthritis of the Thumb," described arthroscopic partial resection of trapezium as well as an interpositional arthroplasty using either autogenous tendon graft, Gore-Tex, or fascia lata allograft as interposed substances. In Menon's paper, it was obvious that the patients had a more advanced stage of arthritis, although his own clinical stages discussed the addition of metacarpal base subluxation as criteria for the stages, and he limited the indications to less than Stage IV disease. In his classification, this correlates to metacarpal base subluxation greater than one third of its diameter and adduction contracture. No mention was made as to whether very early stages of basal joint arthritis were treated with this innovative technique. In fact, the author's hope is to demonstrate that the utility of arthroscopy may be greatest in the earlier stages. The goal of Dr. Menon's groundbreaking technique was to avoid destabilizing the basal joint by avoiding an open arthrotomy to perform hemitrapeziectomy, which had already been described as an open procedure, and interposing the material with the assistance of an arthroscope. Three quarters of the patients had complete pain relief in Menon's series of 25 patients [2]. The results were

comparable to the open technique, but he described several advantages with this minimally invasive technique. For one, it is simply less invasive, and hence has implicit advantages, such as a lesser chance of injuring the radial sensory nerve and decreasing postoperative pain. The less obvious advantage, however, is that arthroscopy of the trapeziometacarpal joint can allow detection of any articular changes long before they would be noted through routine radiographs. This simple fact enables us to treat basal joint osteoarthritis in much earlier stages, and the clinical indication for surgery could simply be pain, not the stage of radiographic disease. This presents a great advantage and allows us to use the arthroscope as a tool for treating younger and more active patients who are in the earliest stages of basal joint arthritis.

One year later in 1997, Richard Berger from the Mayo Clinic in Minnesota presented his experience with thumb CMC joint arthroscopy as a technique paper in the *Journal of Hand Surgery* [3]. Berger felt that small-joint arthroscopic technology presented several advantages over a standard open arthrotomy when joint visualization would be difficult because of the depth of the joint, and opined that one could avoid disruption of the critical ligamentous structures that he so aptly described. After his clear description, he briefly mentioned 12 arthroscopic procedures that he had performed since 1994 with a variety of clinical scenarios, including acute Bennett fractures of the thumb. Berger noted that there was excellent visualization and no complications with this procedure. At that time, the indications for first CMC joint arthroscopy were not clearly defined, but he noted that it was obviously an excellent alternative to arthrotomy for visualizing the anatomy [3]. This paper followed an instructional lecture and demonstration that Berger had performed at the Orthopaedic Learning Center (Rosemont, Illinois) during the wrist arthroscopy course, which the author had the pleasure of attending. Despite its infancy, it was obvious to me at that time that basal joint arthroscopy would have a wide range of application and clinical utility for this common condition. Soon after Berger's landmark paper was published, J. Menon presented a letter to the editor indicating the fact that he had actually published the clinical use of arthroscopy in the basal joint in a previous paper [4]. In Dr. Berger's reply [5], he noted that his technique was developed independently because it was presented as an instructional course in 1995, and the common delay in publication led to this overlap with Dr. Menon's publication. It is clear that both of these authors have made an invaluable contribution to our treatment armamentarium for the basal joint. Further clinical utility was validated in the paper by Osterman and Culp presented in *Arthroscopy* in 1997 [6], in which they defined two groups of patients—traumatic and degenerative—who would benefit from the use of this imaging technology. They, too, felt it had a promising place in the treatment of both acute and chronic conditions of the thumb CMC joint. They were the first to mention that arthroscopy may allow for appropriate staging of the degree of trapezial involvement and may have particular application in the younger patient.

Hence, it is obvious that arthroscopy of the thumb CMC joint allows us to appropriately stage the extent of cartilage degeneration and subsequently determine therapeutic options. The author maintains that the arthroscope can be used not only for treatment of earlier stages but also in advanced stages, as J. Menon so well described [2].

The goals of this article are to describe an arthroscopic classification of the thumb CMC joint and to present a treatment algorithm based upon this staging system. Whether the clinician decides to use arthroscopy definitively for treatment remains an option. Before we expand on the disease staging that arthroscopy allows, we must better understand the ligamentous anatomy and its functional significance as related to biomechanics; however, there can be no argument that the arthroscope gives us the true extent of basal joint disease for the first time.

Functional anatomy

Arthroscopy of the thumb CMC joint has little relevance if the treating surgeon does not understand the ligamentous anatomy. This has been described extensively through cadaver dissections, and over time we will be able to better correlate these open landmarks with the arthroscopic findings. The pioneering description of the trapeziometacarpal ligaments dates way back to 1742, when Weitbrecht described these ligaments in a rudimentary fashion in his book *Syndesmology* [7], reprinted in 1969. Since then, a variety of authors have further described the details of this anatomy, with the most detailed work coming from Bettinger and colleagues at the Mayo Clinic in their 1999 paper [8]. They described a total of 16 ligaments, including ligaments between the metacarpal and trapezium, as well as two ligaments attaching the trapezium to the second metacarpal, and separate stabilizers for the scaphotrapezial and trapezoidal joints. It was their conclusion that this complex of ligaments function as tension bands to prevent instability from cantilever bending forces placed upon the trapezium by the act of pinch [8]. This was a critical concept, because extremely large loads are transferred to the trapezium, and there is no fixed base of support because the scaphoid is an extremely mobile carpal bone. It is the attenuation and pathologic function of these ligaments that may indeed lead to the common scenario of basal joint arthritis. Based upon improved ligamentous understanding, Van Brenk and coworkers [9] suggested that the dorsoradial collateral ligament was in fact the most important ligament in the prevention of trapeziometacarpal subluxation. This was determined by a cadaveric study in which serial sectioning of four separate ligaments determined that the radial collateral ligament (RCL) was the most critical in preventing dorsoradial subluxation [9]. Zancolli and Cozzi, in their landmark *Atlas of Surgical Anatomy of the Hand* [10], supported this concept, but also added the controversial premise that aberrant slips of the abductor pollicis longus (APL) may cause an excessive compressive force of the dorsoradial aspect of trapeziometacarpal (TMC) joint, leading to arthrosis [10]. They felt that the underlying ligamentous laxity may be caused by underlying variations in an individual person's ligamentous laxity, or by a hormonal predisposition that may explain the increased incidence in the female gender. These theories lead to a greater understanding of the causes of basal joint arthritis, and in the future arthroscopic visualization may lend further credence to these theories. Xu and coworkers [11] indicated that the trapeziometacarpal joint is smaller and less congruous in women, and may also have a thinner layer of hyaline cartilage, suggesting that this is a cause for the higher incidence of basal joint osteoarthritis in women. This is the author's experience as well, and suggests that the greatest applicability of arthroscopy may be in younger women who present who have this disease at a much earlier age, and, for whom fewer surgical treatment options exist.

In 1979 in *Hand Clinics*, Pellegrini [12] continued to affirm the biomechanical role that the volar beak ligament plays in preventing dorsal translation of the metacarpal during common functional activities. This ligament and the dorsoradial ligament (DRL), are clearly visualized via arthroscopy, and direct intervention is now feasible. Pellegrini's hypothesis is that there are attritional changes in the beak ligament at the metacarpal insertion site, and that this insertion zone may be particularly sensitive to estrogen-type compounds [12]. This lends further support to the genetic predisposition of this condition. Arthroscopically, the author has also noted particular cartilage loss at the insertion of the volar beak ligament on the deep metacarpal base in the early stages, when the remainder of the hyaline cartilage appears normal. Many of these anatomic, clinical, and biomechanical concepts have been further defined by Bettinger and Berger in their work on the functional ligamentous anatomy of this joint [13]. They did note that the arthroscopic anatomy is much less complicated because only a limited number of structures are able to be seen from the interior perspective. For the first time, they outlined which of the two common portals would lead to clear visualization of what corresponding ligaments [13]. Although they discussed optimal viewing, the reader should note that the small size of this joint allows one to visualize the majority of the surface simply by a change in the viewing direction and the angulation that the arthroscope is held in. Recently other authors have described new portals to help further define the topographic anatomy of this joint. Orellana and Chow [14] described a radial portal that they found was safer because of its proximity to the radial artery and branch of the superficial radial nerve. For this reason, Walsh and colleagues [15] also described another portal, the thenar portal, which was much more volar, actually passing through the thenar muscles to allow for improved triangulation and visualization of the joint via a presumably safer location. These newer portals confirm that thumb CMC arthroscopic surgery is in a state of evolution, and hopefully will allow us to better understand arthritis at this level. A further advantage of this portal is that it does not violate the deep, anterior oblique ligament, which Walsh and colleagues, like Bettinger and Berger [13], feel serves as the major restraining structure against dorsal subluxation. This is in contrast to the biomechanical studies performed by Van Brenk and colleagues [9]. Again, careful documentation of these structures over time may allow arthroscopy to further elucidate the cause of dorsal subluxation as a factor in basal joint arthritis.

Culp and Rekant [16] were the first clinicians to suggest that arthroscopic evaluation, debridement, and synovectomy "offer an exciting alternative for patients who have Eaton and Littler Stages I and II arthritis." They described radiofrequency "painting" of the capsule of the TMC joint to stabilize the critical volar ligaments that may cause dorsal subluxation, and hence arthrosis of the basal joint. They also mention that if the majority of the trapezial surface is abnormal, then at least one-half of the distal trapezium should be resected with an arthroscopic burr [16]. This indicates that a more advanced stage of arthrosis is present, and does not necessarily support its use in the early stages. In fact, their short-term results described in this paper followed arthroscopic hemi- or complete trapeziectomy coupled with electrothermal shrinkage. They had nearly 90% excellent or good outcome in 22 patients with a moderate follow-up. They did make the critical point that no bridges had been burned, because patients who have the arthroscopic procedure can always serve as suitable future candidates for more aggressive complete excisional trapezial arthroplasty by open means. They concluded that debridement and thermal capsular shrinkage is a potentially good treatment for early arthritis of the basal joint [16]. These multiple papers describing the arthroscopic findings make it clear that a more comprehensive staging system is necessary to dictate treatment. All of the clinical results in the studies to date have focused upon more advanced osteoarthritis, and all have discussed the results after an arthroscopic-assisted hemitrapeziectomy. It is perhaps in the patient whose trapezium is largely spared that arthroscopy may find its greatest utility. The author therefore proposes a novel classification to be described herein.

Indications for basal joint arthroscopy

In the author's practice, the vast majority of patients who have the diagnosis of thumb basal joint arthritis who did not improve after conservative treatment underwent arthroscopy for further evaluation of the joint status and surgical treatment during the past 10 years. The disease was staged radiographically according to Eaton's criteria (Table 1) [17]. The notable exceptions were in patients who had advanced Eaton Stage IV arthritis, who then underwent a trapezial excisional suspensionplasty using a slip of abductor pollicus longus. Stage IV patients who had only mild scapho-trapezio-trapezoidal joint (STT) changes were still treated via arthroscopy. Another exception occurred in much older, low-demand patients

Table 1
Proposed Badia arthroscopic classification of thumb trapeziometacarpal osteoarthritis

Stage	Arthroscopic changes
I	Intact articular cartilage Disruption of the dorsoradial ligament and diffuse synovial hypertrophy Inconsistent attenuation of the anterior oblique ligament (AOL)
II	Frank eburnation of the articular cartilage on the ulnar third of the base of first metacarpal and central third of the distal surface of the trapezium Disruption of the dorsoradial ligament + more intense synovial hypertrophy Constant attenuation of the AOL
III	Widespread, full-thickness cartilage loss with or without a peripheral rim on both articular surfaces Less severe synovitis Frayed volar ligaments with laxity

who did well using a cemented total joint arthroplasty, because this required almost no immobilization and minimal therapy. Many of these patients displayed an adduction contracture, and the open arthroplasty permitted an adductor release and a metacarpophalangeal (MCP) joint volar capsulodesis was often needed in cases of severe swan-neck deformity. The last exception was the rare young, male laborer who underwent a TMC joint arthrodesis. This indication has been well-substantiated in the literature [18].

Surgical technique

The arthroscopic procedure is performed under regional anesthesia with tourniquet control. A single Chinese finger trap is used on the thumb with 5 to 8 lbs of longitudinal traction. A shoulder holder, rather than traction tower, is used to more easily facilitate fluoroscopic intervention. The TMC joint is then detected by palpation. The incision for the 1-R (radial) portal, which is used for proper assessment of the DRL, posterior oblique ligament (POL) and ulnar collateral ligament (UCL), is placed just radial to the APL tendon. The incision for the 1-U (ulnar) portal, which allows better evaluation of the anterior oblique ligament (AOL) and UCL, is made just ulnar to the extensor pollicis longus (EPL) tendon. Joint distension is achieved by injecting 2 to 5 mL of normal saline. A short-barrel, 1.9 mm, 30° inclination arthroscope is used for complete visualization of the TMC joint surfaces, capsule,

and ligaments, and then appropriate management is performed as dictated by the pathology found. A full-radius mechanical shaver with suction is used in all cases, particularly for initial debridement and visualization. Many cases are augmented with radiofrequency ablation to perform a more thorough synovectomy. This technology and clinical applications are later expanded upon. Radiofrequency is also used to perform chondroplasty in cases with focal articular cartilage wear or fibrillation. Ligamentous laxity and capsular attenuation are treated with thermal capsulorraphy, also using a radiofrequency shrinkage probe. The author and colleagues are careful to avoid thermal necrosis, and therefore a striping technique is used to tighten the capsule of lax joints. Although the use of radiofrequency is relatively new, we can gain further understanding by prior basic science studies and the clinical application in other joints.

Radiofrequency effects on collagen

Orthopedic surgeons have benefited from the use of radiofrequency in a variety of procedures during the past decade. It is only now that we are realizing that there may be some detrimental effects, and it is important to look at this technology more critically. Nevertheless, as with any new technique, judicious use of this technology may allow for stabilization of the joint capsule in a variety of clinical scenarios. Shoulder instability has been treated by a variety of authors using radiofrequency to stabilize the joint, particularly in those patients who have global instability and who classically have not been considered good operative candidates. It has also been used extensively in the knee, but there has been minimal mention in the literature of its application in the joints of the hand. Obviously this is coupled with the fact that reports on arthroscopy of the TMC joint and the MCP joint have been scant in literature.

Radiofrequency has had many medical applications since its initial use in the 1800s for creating lesions in brain tissue. It has also been used in cardiology, oncology, and colorectal surgery. Lopez and colleagues [19] first demonstrated the effect of radiofrequency energy on the ultrastructure of joint capsular collagen in a histologic study thus titled. They noted that similar applications had been used with a nonablative laser energy in orthopedics, but that radiofrequency offered several advantages over the use of a laser. Not only is it less expensive and safer, but these units are much smaller and easily maneuverable in their application to arthroscopic techniques. Initial studies on a sheep joint indicated that the thermal effect was characterized by the fusion of collagen fibers without tissue ablation, charring, or even crater formation. There was a linear relationship between the degree of collagen fiber fusion and increasing treatment temperature. This indicates that the technology must be treated with respect with avoidance of aggressive use. It was postulated that the coagulated tissue mediates a mild inflammatory reaction that leads to the degradation and replacement of the affected capsule with a denser tissue [19]. This would obviously help to stabilize the joint, and thus would have particular application in the TMC joint based upon previous discussions in this article. In a later study, Hecht and coworkers [20] also looked specifically at the monopolar radiofrequency energy on the joint capsular properties. They concluded that monopolar radiofrequency caused increased capsular damage in the immediate area and depth that correlated with the wattage used. The heat production increased linearly with the duration of application. The arthroscopic lavage could protect the synovial layer from permanent damage as seen in sheep [20]. These findings suggest that radiofrequency probes must be used with adequate fluid lavage as well as for short durations, and with the minimal wattage necessary to achieve the desired effect. The author refers specifically to monopolar radiofrequency because it is a common understanding amongst orthopedic surgeons that monopolar radiofrequency causes less heat production than bipolar modalities. This is particularly important to the hand surgeon, because there are close neurovascular structures directly overlying the joint capsule in the small joints as compared with the knee or shoulder. Further understanding may be gleaned in the future if a direct clinical comparison can be made with monopolar versus bipolar radiofrequency treatments in the small joints.

Arthroscopic staging

Arthroscopic Stage I patients are characterized by diffuse synovitis, but with minimal, if any, articular cartilage loss (Fig. 1). Ligamentous laxity, particularly the entire volar capsule, is a frequent finding. This presentation is relatively uncommon, because most patients present late, having suffered with symptoms for a long period; or are referred at

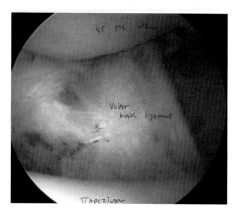

Fig. 1. Arthroscopic Stage I findings demonstrate synovitis around the volar oblique ligament, with intact articular cartilage on the trapezium.

a delayed time once conservative means have been exhausted. These patients undergo synovectomy, both mechanical and by radiofrequency, with occasional shrinkage capsulorraphy performed, depending on findings. The joint is then protected in a thumb spica cast from 1 to 4 weeks, depending on the extent of capsular laxity. More unstable joints required longer immobilization to achieve joint stability and presumably slow the progression of articular cartilage degeneration.

Arthroscopic Stage II patients are characterized by focal wear of the articular surface on the central to dorsal aspect of the trapezium. In the author's mind, this represents an irreversible process, and requires a joint-modifying procedure to alter the vector force across the joint. After synovectomy, debridement, and occasional loose body removal, the joint is reassessed to determine the extent of instability and capsular attenuation (Fig. 2). A shrinkage thermal capsulorraphy is performed in many of the cases, with chondroplasty frequently performed to anneal the cartilage borders (Fig. 3). The arthroscope is then removed and the ulnar portal extended distally to expose the metacarpal base. A dorsoradial closing wedge osteotomy, similar to Wilson's original technique [21], is then performed to place the thumb in a more extended and abducted position. This is to minimize the tendency for metacarpal subluxation and to change the contact points of worn articular cartilage. The osteotomy is protected by a single oblique Kirschner wire that is also placed across the first CMC joint in a reduced position.

This allows for healing of the osteotomy in the correct position, and also a correction of the

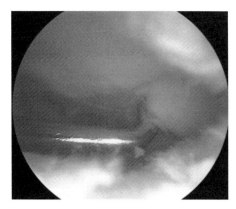

Fig. 2. Arthroscopic Stage II typical findings include small area of articular cartilage loss on deep aspect of metacarpal at insertion of volar beak ligament and central, focal loss of trapezial joint surface. This stage often demonstrates loose bodies as seen here during extrication.

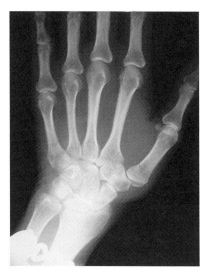

Fig. 4. Preoperative radiograph in middle-aged woman demonstrating metacarpal base subluxation free of osteophytes. Arthroscopy demonstrated focal trapezial wear indicative of Badia arthroscopic Stage II arthritis. Patient indicated for osteotomy of metacarpal base.

metacarpal subluxation often seen in this stage. A thumb spica cast protects this during healing, and the wire is removed at 5 weeks postoperative. Only arthroscopy can determine the optimal indications for this osteotomy, which has demonstrated good results in the past, and in a more recent paper by Tomaino [22]. Late follow up on the author's patients has demonstrated that the metacarpal remains "centralized," and it is unclear if the capsular shrinkage plays a role versus the alteration of biomechanics by the use of osteotomy (Figs. 4 and 5).

Arthroscopic Stage III is characterized by much more diffuse trapezial articular cartilage

loss (Fig. 6). The metacarpal base can also be devoid of cartilage to varying degrees. Arthroscopic findings indicate that this is not a joint worth preserving, and a simple debridement or even accompanying osteotomy will not give a good long-term

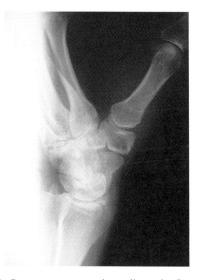

Fig. 5. One-year postoperative radiograph after metacarpal osteotomy (and pin removal) demonstrating the persistent "centralization" of the metacarpal on the trapezium. This changes the joint contact points that may have led to progression of arthrosis and pain.

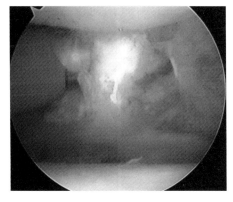

Fig. 3. Shrinkage capsulorraphy being performed on deep aspect of capsule noted to be attenuated because of chronic deposition of corticosteroid.

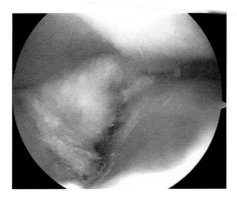

Fig. 6. Arthroscopic Stage III findings include diffuse articular cartilage loss on both trapezium and metacarpal base. Chronic inflammation leads to capsular fraying evident here.

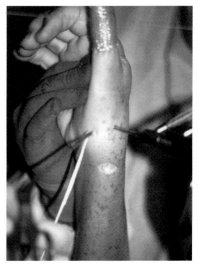

Fig. 7. External view of thumb base denoting the traction method and ulnar portal placement of the arthroscope with APL tendon slip insertion via the radial portal.

result in this case. An arthroscopic hemitrapeziectomy is then performed by burring away the remaining articular cartilage and also removing subchondral bone down to a bleeding surface. This serves to not only increase the joint space, but to allow for bleeding that will form an organized thrombus, which will adhere to an interposed tendon graft. This graft, either palmaris longus or the volar slip of APL, is inserted via a portal, similar to the technique as proposed by Menon [2] (Fig. 7). A thumb spica cast in an abducted position is then maintained for 4 weeks, followed by hand therapy to focus on pinch strengthening. Stage III can also be treated by a traditional open excisional arthroplasty [23–26], arthrodesis [18], or total joint replacement [27], depending on surgeon preference.

Arthroscopic/radiographic correlation

The most consistent arthroscopic findings in the group of patients who display radiographic changes compatible with Stage I of the disease include fibrillation of the articular cartilage on the ulnar third of the base of the first metacarpal, disruption of the dorsoradial ligament, and diffuse synovial hypertrophy (see Fig. 1). A less reliable discovery is attenuation of the POL.

Regular arthroscopic findings noted in patients classified as having Stage II arthritis include frank eburnation of the articular cartilage of the ulnar third of the metacarpal base and central third of the distal surface of the trapezium, disruption of the DRL, more noticeable attenuation of the POL, and more intense synovial hypertrophy (see Figs. 2 and 3). Most of the patients in this

arthroscopic stage also presented radiographically as Stage II, but on occasion patients deemed Stage I may actually have more advanced findings once the joint is truly assessed. Herein lies one of the great advantages of this technology. Only the rare case demonstrates less cartilage wear than supposed on the plain film. Consequently, radiographic Stage III rarely is considered Stage II, but that does greatly influence and expand the treatment options. Because this stage may have the most clinical impact on our method of treatment, due to lack of good options, it is important to review the patient outcomes for arthroscopic Stage II disease.

Preliminary Stage II results

A retrospective assessment evaluated arthroscopic Stage II patients with adequate follow-up in a selected 3-year period. Forty-three patients (38 female and 5 male) were arthroscopically diagnosed as having Stage II basal joint osteoarthritis of the thumb between 1998 and 2001. All the procedures were performed by the author, with follow-up data generated by visiting fellows for objectivity. The average patient age was 51 (range: 31–69). The right thumb was involved in 23 patients and the left in 20. There was no improvement after a minimum 6 weeks of conservative treatment under the author's direction. The surgical procedure consisted of arthroscopic synovectomy, debridement, and occasional thermal capsulorraphy, followed by an extension-abduction closing wedge osteotomy in all cases. A 0.045-inch Kirschner wire provided stability to the osteotomy site, and a short arm-thumb spica cast was used for 4 to 6 weeks until pin removal. The average follow-up was 43 months (range: 24–64 months).

Consistent arthroscopic findings in the selected group were frank eburnation of the articular cartilage of the ulnar third of the base of the first metacarpal and central third of the distal surface of the trapezium, disruption of the dorsoradial ligament, attenuation of the anterior oblique ligament, and synovial hypertrophy. The osteotomy healed within 4 to 6 weeks in all the cases. Radiographic studies at final follow-up depicted maintenance of centralization of the metacarpal base over the trapezium and no progression of arthritic changes in 42 patients. Average range of thumb MCP joint motion was 5° to 50°, and thumb opposition reached the base of the small finger in all cases. The average pinch strength was 9.5 lbs (73% from nonaffected side). At final follow-up, 37 patients had no pain, 3 had mild pain, 2 had moderate pain, and the only patient who complained of severe pain had undergone arthroscopic-assisted hemitrapeziectomy because of progressive arthritis. These preliminary results suggest that continued use of this technique is appropriate. A longer follow-up will be later obtained to better assess the long-term utility of this technique and to publish these findings specifically in Stage II patients.

Arthroscopy in patients who had radiographic features of Stage III and IV generally displays widespread full thickness cartilage loss, with or without a peripheral rim on both articular surfaces, severe synovitis; and frayed volar ligaments with laxity (see Figs. 4 and 5). This clearly constitutes arthroscopic Stage III, and the treatment options here are quite varied. The arthroscope can be removed and the most appropriate open procedure performed, or as the author prefers in most cases, an arthroscopic interposition arthroplasty is undertaken.

Based on the above findings and clinical experience, the author proposes the arthroscopic classification and treatment algorithm delineated in Table 1 and Fig. 8.

Discussion

Clinical assessment and radiographic studies used to be the only tools available for the selection of treatment modalities for thumb CMC arthritis [28,29]. Eaton and Glickel proposed a staging system for this disease that has been widely applied [17]. Later, Bettinger and coworkers [30] described the trapezial tilt as an instrument to predict further progression of the disease. They found that in advanced Stages (Eaton III and IV) the trapezial tilt was high (50° ± 4°; normal: 42° ± 4°). Barron and Eaton [31] concluded that there appears to be no indication for MRI, tomography, or ultrasonography in the routine evaluation of basal joint disease .

Although the author believes that a radiographic classification is important for a stepwise interpretation of the progression of this entity, my experience has demonstrated instances when it is very difficult to make an accurate diagnosis of the extent of disease based solely on radiographic studies. Recent advances in arthroscopic technology have allowed complete examination of smaller joints throughout the body with minimal morbidity [1]. Moreover, arthroscopy has already proved to be reliable for direct evaluation of the first CMC joint, as previously discussed [3].

In early stages of thumb basal joint arthritis, in Eaton Stage I, for instance, it is very common to find essentially normal radiographic studies despite the presence of painful limitation of the thumb. In the experience of the author and coworkers, this group of patients displays mild to moderate synovitis that could benefit from a thorough joint debridement combined with thermal shrinkage of the ligaments to enhance the stability. This, of course, assumes that they have not responded well to conservative treatment, including splinting, use of nonsteroidal anti-inflammatory drugs (NSAIDs), and corticosteroid injection. This stage is typically seen in middle-aged women who tend not to be indicated for more aggressive open procedures [29]. Arthroscopic treatment provides a particularly good option for this ubiquitous subset of patients.

Tomaino [22] concluded that first metacarpal extension osteotomy is a good treatment option for Eaton Stage I. This may not be necessary in the occasional patient who undergoes arthroscopy at an early time and demonstrates no focal cartilage loss. Future studies may indicate that synovectomy, and perhaps thermal capsulorraphy, may avoid progression of disease and the need for a mechanical intervention; however, the arthroscopic findings that the author previously described for arthroscopic Stage II of the disease

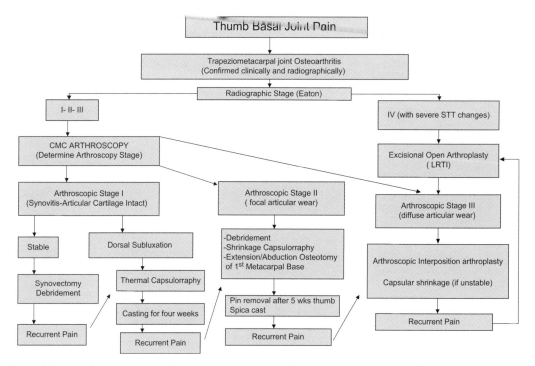

Fig. 8. Schematic for management of trapeziometacarpal arthritis, incorporating arthroscopic stages and subsequent treatment decision-making. LRTI, ligament reconstruction tendon interposition.

demand a joint modification such as osteotomy, to minimize the chance of further articular degeneration. My retrospective study indicates that this approach is efficacious, with only one out of 43 thumbs developing progressive arthritis requiring further surgery.

There is no doubt that if complete articular cartilage loss is the arthroscopic scenario, then the logical further step is to perform some type of trapezium excision with interposition arthroplasty. This can include either a partial or complete excision or replacement. Menon [2] described a technique demonstrating arthroscopic debridement of the trapezial articular surface and interposition of autogenous tendon, fascia lata, or Gore-Tex patch into the CMC joint in patients who had Stage II and III, with excellent results. Newer techniques may allow the arthroscopic insertion of Artelon (Small Bone Innovations, New York, New York), which has proven successful with open techniques and confirmed histologically [32]. In either case, complete excision of the trapezium may not be desirable or even necessary, particularly in younger patients. This Stage III treatment needs to be further assessed by evaluating long-term clinical results.

According to the arthroscopic classification proposed, the author recommends arthroscopic synovectomy and debridement of the basal joint in patients who have Stage I arthritis. In patients who have Stage II disease, synovectomy and debridement is combined with osteotomy of the first metacarpal. In both these stages, thermal shrinkage is used to manage ligamentous laxity. Finally, for Stage III of the disease, arthroscopic interposition arthroplasty is my treatment of choice, although other factors must be considered in making this determination.

Summary

Arthroscopic assessment of the CMC joint allows direct visualization of all components of the joint, including synovium, articular surfaces, ligaments, and the joint capsule. It also allows for the extent of joint pathology to be evaluated and staged with intraoperative management decisions made based on this information. The author recommends this arthroscopic staging to ensure better judgment of this condition in order to provide the most adequate treatment option to patients who have this disabling condition.

Future studies assessing the clinical long term results using arthroscopy will likely ensure its place in the treatment armamentarium for trapeziometacarpal osteoarthritis.

References

[1] Chen YC. Arthroscopy of the wrist and finger joints. Orthop Clin North Am 1979;10:723–33.

[2] Menon J. Arthroscopic management of trapeziometacarpal joint arthritis of the thumb. Arthroscopy 1996;12:581–7.

[3] Berger RA. Technique for arthroscopic evaluation of the first carpometacarpal joint. J Hand Surg [Am] 1997;22:1077–80.

[4] Menon J. Arthroscopic evaluation of the first carpometacarpal joint [letter to the editor]. J Hand Surg [Am] 1998;23:757.

[5] Berger R. Arthroscopic evaluation of the first carpometacarpal joint [reply to letter to the editor]. J Hand Surg [Am] 1998;23:757.

[6] Osterman AL, Culp R, Bednar J. Arthroscopy of the thumb carpometacarpal joint. Arthroscopy 1997;13:411.

[7] Weitbrecht J. Syndesmology (1742). Philadelphia: WB Saunders; 1969.

[8] Bettinger PC, Linscheid RL, Berger RA, et al. An anatomic study of the stabilizing ligaments of the trapezium and trapeziometacarpal joint. J Hand Surg [Am] 1999;24:786–98.

[9] Van Brenk B, Richards RR, Mackay MB, et al. A biomechanical assessment of ligaments preventing dorsoradial subluxation of the trapeziometacarpal joint. J Hand Surg [Am] 1998;23:607–11.

[10] Zancolli EA, Cozzi EP. The trapeziometacarpal joint: anatomy and mechanics. In: Zancolli E, Cozzi EP, editors. Atlas of surgical anatomy of the hand. New York: Churchill Livingstone; 1992. p. 443–4.

[11] Xu L, Strauch RJ, Ateshian GA, et al. Topography of the osteoarthritic thumb carpometacarpal joint and its variation with regard to gender, age, site, and osteoarthritic stage. J Hand Surg [Am] 1998;23:454–65.

[12] Pelligrini VD. Pathomechanics of the thumb trapeziometacarpal joint. Hand Clin 2001;17:175–84.

[13] Bettinger PC, Berger RA. Functional ligamentous anatomy of the trapezium and trapeziometacarpal joint (gross and arthroscopic). Hand Clin 2001;17(2):151–69.

[14] Orellana MA, Chow JC. Arthroscopic visualization of the thumb carpometacarpal joint: introduction and evaluation of a new radial portal. Arthroscopy 2003;19(6):583–91.

[15] Walsh EF, Akelman E, Fleming BC, et al. Thumb carpometacarpal arthroscopy: a topographic, anatomic study of the thenar portal. J Hand Surg [Am] 2005;30:373–9.

[16] Culp RW, Rekant MS. The role of arthroscopy in evaluating and treating trapeziometacarpal disease. Hand Clin 2001;17(2):315–9.

[17] Eaton RG, Glickel SZ. Trapeziometacarpal osteoarthritis. Staging as a rationale for treatment. Hand Clin 1987;3:455–71.

[18] Fulton DB, Stern PJ. Trapeziometacarpal arthrodesis in primary osteoarthritis: a minimum two year follow-up study. J Hand Surg [Am] 2001;26:109–14.

[19] Lopez MJ, Hayashi K, Fanton GS, et al. The effects of radiofrequency energy on the ultrastructure of joint capsular collagen. Arthroscopy 1998;14(5):495–501.

[20] Hecht P, Hayashi K, Cooley AJ, et al. The thermal effect of monopolar radiofrequency energy on the properties of joint capsule. Am J Sports Med 1998;26(6):808–14.

[21] Wilson J. Osteotomy of the first metacarpal in the treatment of arthritis of the carpometacarpal joint of the thumb. Br J Surg 1973;60:854–8.

[22] Tomaino MM. Treatment of Eaton Stage I trapeziometacarpal disease. Ligament reconstruction or thumb metacarpal extension osteotomy? Hand Clin 2001;17:197–205.

[23] Eaton RG, Glickel SZ, Littler JW. Tendon interposition arthroplasty for degenerative arthritis of the trapeziometacarpal joint of the thumb. J Hand Surg [Am] 1985;10:645–54.

[24] Burton RI, Pellegrini VD Jr. Surgical management of basal joint arthritis of the thumb: Part II. Ligament reconstruction with tendon interposition arthroplasty. J Hand Surg [Am] 1986;11:324–32.

[25] Tomaino MM, Pellegrini VD Jr, Burton RI. Arthroplasty of the basal joint of the thumb: long-term follow-up after ligament reconstruction with tendon interposition. J Bone Joint Surg 1995;77A:346–55.

[26] Lins RE, Gelberman RH, McKeown L, et al. Basal joint arthritis: trapeziectomy with ligament reconstruction and tendon interposition arthroplasty. J hand Surg [Am] 1996;21:202–9.

[27] Braun RM. Total joint replacement at the base of the thumb—preliminary report. J Hand Surg 1982;7:245–51.

[28] Froimson AI. Tendon arthroplasty of the trapeziometacarpal joint. Clin Orthop 1970;70:191–9.

[29] Swigart CR, Eaton RG, Glickel SZ. Splinting in the treatment of arthritis of the first carpometacarpal joint. J Hand Surg [Am] 1999;24:86–91.

[30] Bettinger PC, Linscheid RL, Cooney WP 3rd, et al. Trapezial tilt: a radiographic correlation with advanced trapeziometacarpal joint arthritis. J Hand Surg [Am] 2001;26:692–7.

[31] Barron OA, Eaton RG. Save the trapezium: double interposition arthroplasty for the treatment of Stage IV disease of the basal joint. J Hand Surg [Am] 1998;23:196–204.

[32] Nilsson A, Liljensten E. Results from a degradable TMC joint spacer (Artelon) compared with tendon arthroplasty. J Hand Surg [Am] 2005;30:380–9.

Trapeziectomy

John D. Mahoney, MD, Roy A. Meals, MD*

*Combined Orthopaedic and Plastic Surgery Hand Service, University of California, Los Angeles,
100 UCLA Medical Plaza, #305, Los Angeles, CA 90024, USA*

Primary osteoarthritis of the carpometacarpal joint of the thumb is a common problem, especially in women beyond the fifth decade. Patients usually present with activity-related pain at the base of the thumb. The usual first line of treatment may include activity modification, pain-relieving medications, splinting, and possibly corticosteroid injections. When these nonoperative measures have failed to preserve or restore the patient's quality of life, surgical intervention may be appropriate.

Many different surgical alternatives are described for the treatment of thumb carpometacarpal joint arthritis, and most begin with at least partial trapeziectomy. The first description of simple trapeziectomy was by Gervis in 1949 [1]. He reported good pain relief, but later publications on trapeziectomy by Murley [2] and Iyer [3] noted substantial weakness, which was assumed to be caused by instability at the base of the metacarpal. In all of these patients, no suspension of the thumb metacarpal was performed to prevent subsidence, and the patients were started on an immediate motion protocol postoperatively.

To improve the stability of the thumb carpometacarpal joint and thereby the strength of the hand, Eaton and Littler in 1973 [4] first described volar oblique ligament reconstruction. This report was followed by Burton and Pellegrini's report in 1986 [5] of ligament reconstruction and tendon interposition. These techniques were based on three essential components to reconstruct the thumb carpometacarpal joint: (1) reconstruction of the volar oblique ligament, (2) interposition of tendon graft into the space formerly occupied by the trapezium, and (3) temporary fixation of the thumb metacarpal base to the adjacent index metacarpal [6]. The results of these more complicated techniques were generally excellent.

Subsequent reports have questioned the necessity of each of these components. Trapeziectomy alone, tendon interposition without ligament reconstruction, and ligament reconstruction without tendon interposition have each been reported to result in satisfactory outcome. In fact, a recent prospective, randomized controlled study by Davis and colleagues [7] found that trapeziectomy and Kirschner wire (K-wire) fixation was as effective as ligament reconstruction and placement of a soft-tissue spacer.

The authors believe that simple trapeziectomy with hematoma and distraction arthroplasty is as effective as more complicated procedures. Although it may seem unsettling to remove the trapezium and not replace it with something, or to leave the body to its own devices to reform a functional beak ligament, we know that the body has remarkable capacities to heal itself. The act of trapeziectomy may incite enough sterile commotion to allow a vigorous scar bed to fill in the site of the trapezium. Thus, the base of the thumb metacarpal is held at bay from the scaphoid by this cushion of scar, providing the same benefits of interposition arthroplasty with foreign material without the potential complications.

Surgical technique

Trapeziectomy and hematoma distraction arthroplasty of the thumb carpometacarpal joint is indicated in both inflammatory and degenerative arthritis that has failed conservative management.

* Corresponding author.
E-mail address: rmeals@ucla.edu (R.A. Meals).

0749-0712/06/$ - see front matter © 2006 Elsevier Inc. All rights reserved.
doi:10.1016/j.hcl.2006.02.003

When necessary, the procedure is combined with volar plate capsulodesis of the thumb metacarpophalangeal joint to correct hyperextension. The procedure may be performed under regional block or general anesthesia. The usual operative time for hematoma distraction arthroplasty alone is approximately 35 minutes.

A curved, dorsal radial incision is made over the carpometacarpal joint of the thumb. Sharp dissection is made through the skin only. Blunt subcutaneous dissection is made down to the first dorsal compartment. The branches of the radial sensory nerve are retracted out of the operative field. Blunt dissection then proceeds ulnarly and dorsally from the first dorsal compartment over the capsule of the trapezium until the radial artery is encountered. Dissection between the radial artery and the underlying joint capsule will allow retraction of the artery safely out of the way.

With the radial artery and the branches of the radial sensory nerve safely retracted, the base of the thumb metacarpal is palpated and the carpometacarpal joint is identified. A longitudinal capsular incision is made just ulnar and dorsal to the tendons of the first dorsal compartment. The incision begins 5 mm on the base of the metacarpal, and is carried proximally until the scapho-trapezial joint is encountered. The capsule is elevated radially and ulnarly off of the base of the metacarpal and the trapezium. Occasionally, in cases of severe subluxation, the trapezium may be difficult to palpate, and even after capsular incision may be difficult to see. Longitudinal

traction on the thumb will distract the joint and allow visual confirmation of the various carpal bones.

Before excision, the trapezium should be definitively confirmed by inspection of the saddle joint and the base of the metacarpal. If there is any doubt, an intraoperative radiograph can be used with a Freer elevator placed into what the surgeon believes is the carpometacarpal joint.

The trapezium is removed piecemeal. The trapezium is first divided longitudinally with an osteotome into three or four pieces. A rongeur, an elevator, and a knife can then be used to free the pieces of the trapezium from the investing capsule. The flexor carpi radialis and flexor pollicis longus tendons must be protected at the base of the wound. The surgeon's finger can be introduced into the wound to palpate for small fragments of bone that may be painful later. These fragments are most commonly in the volar aspect of the wound.

Once the trapezium is removed, the wound is irrigated and the thumb is set for distraction and fixation. The thumb is grasped and held in a position of wide palmar abduction, slight opposition, and distraction until firm resistance is felt. A single 1.6 mm (0.062″) K-wire is inserted percutaneously from the base of the thumb metacarpal in a transverse orientation to anchor into the base of the index metacarpal or into the trapezoid (Fig. 1). A second K-wire may be used to provide additional stability. The wire is cut above the skin. Although transverse placement

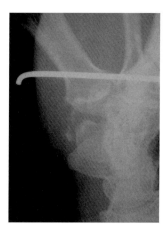
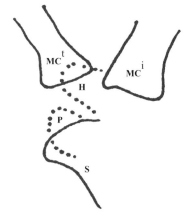

Fig. 1. Postoperative radiograph showing proper position of K-wire fixation after hematoma and distraction arthroplasty. H, hamate; MC^i, index finger metacarpal; MC^t, thumb metacarpal; P, pisiform; S, scaphoid. (*From* Kuhns CA, Emerson ET, Meals RA. Hematoma and distraction arthroplasty for thumb basal joint osteoarthritis: a prospective, single-surgeon study including outcome measures. J Hand Surg 2003;28A:381–9; with permission.)

of the K-wire risks antegrade migration and dorsal hand pain or even ulceration, the authors prefer this to longitudinal K-wire placement, because the thumb metacarpal may slide proximally along the longitudinally-oriented K-wire and close the trapezial void before a dense hematoma and fibroblastic scar can form.

The dorsal capsular remnants are closed to the extent possible. After skin closure, a thumb spica splint is fit to the hand and wrist, with care taken to relieve any pressure from the splint against the trailing end of the K-wire. The sutures are removed at 10 days postoperatively, and a short arm-thumb spica cast is applied, leaving the thumb pulp free for light pinch activities. Again, care is taken with padding the trailing end of the K-wire to preclude pressure against the rigid cast material and subsequent migration. This cast and K-wire are removed 4 weeks later, approximately 5.5 weeks postoperatively. The thumb is protected with a 2″ elastic roller bandage, and the patient is advised to gradually wean from use of the bandage over the next 4 to 5 days, and to begin a home exercise program immediately to regain full adduction and opposition of the thumb. The patient is advised to use the hand as normally as pain and postimmobilization stiffness permit. The patients are seen again 2 weeks later, and those patients that cannot abduct the thumb out from the plane of the hand and touch the tip of the thumb to the small finger metacarpal head are referred to hand therapy for range-of-motion exercises. The therapists are instructed not to perform or instruct in formal strengthening exercises, which have been seen to prolong the inflammatory flare. The authors prefer that the patient gradually recover strength through progressively increasing daily use of the thumb over the first 6 to 12 months after surgery.

Results

The authors' technique has been reported recently [8], with results at a minimum of 2 years showing very favorable relief of pain with good return of function. The majority of patients recover full opposition and full abduction out of the plane of the palm in several weeks without formal hand therapy. Nearly all patients recover full opposition and palmar abduction, and on average, the strengths at 2 years increase over preoperative measurements by 47% for grip, 33% for key pinch, and 23% for tip pinch. Radiographs have

shown that the metacarpal tends to subside toward the scaphoid more than with the procedures that include a formal beak ligament reconstruction. The authors' study as well as others, however, has not showed a relationship between subsidence and pain, strength, or patient satisfaction. In fact, the results of our 2-year follow-up study showed greater recovery of normal motion and greater grip and pinch strengths than reported in the literature for procedures that include a formal ligament reconstruction [8].

To ensure that the hematoma and distraction arthroplasty is entirely durable, the authors are presently conducting a 6- to 8-year follow-up study of the same group of patients, and the early data are equally promising. Anecdotally, the senior author (RM) has been performing the hematoma and distraction arthroplasty for approximately 20 years while practicing in the same location and with the same phone number. During that time, the senior author has not personally revised a hematoma distraction arthroplasty or heard that a revision was needed or performed elsewhere.

Complications

Radial sensory neuritis is occasionally noted postoperatively. This potential complication can be minimized by identification and retraction of the radial sensory nerve branches out of the operative field during the procedure. In the authors' experience, the rare patient that develops radial sensory neuritis can expect full recovery within a year.

K-wire problems include skin irritation around the pin, loosening, and migration. The risk of pin-skin irritation is minimized by releasing undue skin tension around the pin at the time of surgery. Pin track infections are possible, but are rarely encountered. Pin loosening and migration can be prevented with precise placement of the pin within the center axis of each metacarpal; with the wire driver turning at low speed; with as few passes of the pin as possible, just barely penetrating the second cortex of the anchoring bone with only the tip of the K-wire; and with protecting the trailing end of the K-wire against pressure from the overlying splint or cast [9,10]. A loose or migrated pin usually requires early removal. In our reported series [8], early K-wire removal did not cause noted deterioration of results. These patients were still immobilized for the full 5.5 weeks in a short arm-thumb spica cast.

Discussion

Several questions naturally arise. The hematoma and distraction arthroplasty is a slight variation of the simple trapeziectomy procedure from the 1950s that was discarded because of poor results. What is the difference that makes the hematoma and distraction arthroplasty successful? The authors feel that the immobilization of the thumb in a distracted position for 5 to 6 weeks after surgery allows the hematoma to organize, and the surrounding capsular remnants to consolidate to sufficiently anchor the metacarpal base in a secure position, yet allow for recovery of a normal range of motion. To promote the goal of having the body respond to the surgery with a sufficient inflammatory response to generate supporting scar tissue, it may be valuable to remove the trapezium piecemeal using osteotome, elevator and rongeurs. In this manner, capsular tears are expected, and small flakes of trapezium remain attached to the capsular remnants; all well-suited to aid in a florid inflammatory response. Other authors have advised removing the trapezium in one piece using curved knives and perhaps aided by placing a joystick (large, long cancellous screw or screw tap) to turn and twist the trapezium. The authors find removal of the trapezium piecemeal quicker and technically easier, and think that the additional capsular injury thereby inflicted actually promotes more scar formation and the desired degree of metacarpal stability, without the need for a formal beak ligament reconstruction.

If the results are no different when the K-wire has required removal 2 to 4 weeks after surgery than when leaving it the recommended 5.5 weeks, why not routinely remove it earlier? The authors are uncertain of the minimum length of time needed to achieve the distinct improvement in results of the hematoma and distraction arthroplasty, as compared with the simple trapezial excisions reported in the 1950s. Based on the appearance of the surgical site and on the patient's comfort, as well as on general principles of wound healing and collagen deposition and maturation, immobilization of the thumb in a splint or cast for 5 to 6 weeks is appropriate. Because the thumb is to be externally immobilized for that length of time and the presence of the K-wire during that time generally presents no problem, the authors see no benefit in testing the lower limit of time actually needed for the distraction afforded by the K-wire.

If the hematoma and distraction arthroplasty is simpler and faster to perform, and the published results are equal to or superior to the procedures that reconstruct a ligament with or without an interposition into the trapezial void, why is it not universally used?

Intuition leads one to replace broken or worn out parts. Patients and doctors alike have experience with car and dishwasher repairs, for example, and it would be illogical simply to remove and not replace a defective spark plug or gasket. So in explaining surgical options to a patient who has basal joint arthritis, it is easy for the doctor to explain and for the patient to understand when a stretched ligament will be reconstructed and the arthritic bone will be replaced with interposed material. More so for patients, but also true for hand surgeons, we do not routinely give the natural healing capacity of the living body the credit it deserves. For example, surgeons tend to state that we "repair" nerves and tendons, whereas we actually only suture them and biology does the actual repair. In this light, the surgeon and the patient must have confidence that the body can actually restore a naturally and durably stable and mobile thumb base without mechanistically reconstructing prearthritic order. Further long-term follow-up on the hematoma and distraction arthroplasty from multiple centers should enhance confidence that the body does indeed have that needed capacity.

References

[1] Gervis WH. Excision of the trapezium for osteoarthritis of the trapezio-metacarpal joint. J Bone Joint Surg 1949;31B:537–9.
[2] Murley AHG. Excision of the trapezium in osteoarthritis of the first carpo-metacarpal joint. J Bone Joint Surg 1960;42B:502–7.
[3] Iyer KM. The results of excision of the trapezium. Hand 1981;13:198–250.
[4] Eaton RG, Littler JW. Ligament reconstruction for the painful thumb carpometacarpal joint. J Bone Joint Surg 1973;55A:1656–66.
[5] Burton RI, Pellegrini VD Jr. Surgical management of basal joint arthritis of the thumb: Part II. Ligament reconstruction with tendon interposition arthroplasty. J Hand Surg [Am] 1986;11:324–32.
[6] Manske PR. Commentary: excision of the trapezium. J Hand Surg [Am] 2004;29:1078–9.
[7] Davis TRC, Brady O, Dias JJ. Excision of the trapezium for osteoarthritis of the trapeziometacarpal joint: a study of the benefit of ligament

reconstruction or tendon interposition. J Hand Surg [Am] 2004;29:1069–77.

[8] Kuhns CA, Emerson ET, Meals RA. Hematoma and distraction arthroplasty for thumb basal joint osteoarthritis: a prospective, single-surgeon study including outcome measures. J Hand Surg [Am] 2003;28:381–9.

[9] Namba R, Kabo J, Meals R. Biomechanical effects of point configuration in Kirschner wire fixation. Clin Orthop 1987;214:19–22.

[10] Graebe A, Tsenter M, Kabo J, et al. Biomechanical effects of a new point configuration and a modified cross-sectional configuration in Kirschner wire fixation. Clin Orthop 1992;283:292–5.

ELSEVIER
SAUNDERS

Hand Clin 22 (2006) 171–175

HAND
CLINICS

Suspensionplasty for Basal Joint Arthritis: Why and How

Matthew M. Tomaino, MD, MBA

Department of Orthopaedics, Division of Hand, Shoulder and Elbow Surgery,
University of Rochester Medical Center, 601 Elmwood Avenue, Box 665, Rochester, NY 14642, USA

The thumb trapeziometacarpal (TM) joint is the second most commonly involved site of osteoarthritis in the hand, after the distal interphalangeal (DIP) joint, but its involvement potentially causes far more significant functional disability secondary to painful, weakened pinch and grip. Many treatment alternatives exist, and the literature is replete with reports of favorable outcome following TM arthrodesis, trapezium excision alone, in combination with tissue interposition, and in combination with ligament reconstruction. In this report, the author shares the rationale for performing ligament reconstruction (suspensionplasty) at the time of trapezium excision and details how and why his technique has changed since he described the ligament reconstruction tendon interposition (LRTI) arthroplasty in May 2001 in this publication [1].

Rationale for suspensionplasty

The primary rationale for performing suspensionplasty revolves around resisting the sagittal plane collapse that occurs when the thumb is loaded during pinch. In the absence of a volar-based suspension of the metacarpal, cantilever bending forces and axial force transmission result in the dissipation of force along the thumb lever arm [2,3]. In the absence of ligamentous restraint [4], this results in metacarpal adduction and proximal migration. Outcome metrics that focus on pain relief alone do not reveal this, and study designs in published comparisons of trapeziectomy

with and without suspensionplasty have not enabled a valid objective strength comparison between the two alternatives [5].

An appreciation of normal ligamentous anatomy and thumb mechanics, pathomechanics, and pathoanatomy are integral to the author's advocacy of ligament reconstruction at the time of trapeziectomy. The TM joint is a biconcave-convex saddle joint with minimal bony constraints. A pinch force of 1 kg at the thumb tip is magnified up to 13.42 kg at the TM joint [2]; thus, in the absence of ligamentous restraint, substantial cantilever bending forces will cause tangential dorsoradial subluxation.

Bettinger and colleagues [4] have furthered our understanding of ligamentous anatomy with the assistance of TM joint arthroscopy. These authors have described 16 ligaments, some of which function as tension bands to resist cantilever-bending forces of the metacarpal on the trapezium, thus providing a stable base for the TM joint. They have further defined the anterior oblique ligament (AOL) into a superficial (sAOL) and deep ligament (dAOL). The dAOL, which is intracapsular, is in fact the beak ligament, and plays an important role in the kinematics of thumb opposition. It acts as a pivot point, and becomes tight during pronation, opposition, and palmar abduction.

Pathomechanics and pathoanatomy provide additional compelling data in support of ligament restoration following trapeziectomy. Pellegrini [6,7] showed that the primary loading areas during lateral pinch are in the same palmar regions of the joint as the eburnated surfaces in diseased joints. Division of the beak ligament in specimens with healthy cartilage surfaces altered the contact patterns and reproduced the topography of the

E-mail address: matthew_tomaino@urmc.rochester.edu

0749-0712/06/$ - see front matter © 2006 Elsevier Inc. All rights reserved.
doi:10.1016/j.hcl.2006.02.009

eburnated lesions observed in the arthritic joints. Histological study showed that attritional changes in the beak ligament, where it attaches to the palmar lip of the metacarpal, preceded degeneration of cartilage [8].

In summary, degeneration of the beak ligament leads to the development of TM osteoarthritis. Functional incompetence of this palmar ligament results in pathologic laxity, abnormal translation of the metacarpal on the trapezium, and generation of excessive shear forces between the joint surfaces during grip and pinch activity. It only follows, therefore, that its reconstruction seems justified when performing basal joint arthroplasty.

Additional advocacy on behalf of suspensionplasty

Advanced basal joint disease implies end-stage degeneration of the TM joint (stages 2–4), salvageable only by a procedure that removes or replaces the entire articular surface. Although TM fusion provides superlative pain relief and outcomes potentially comparable to ligament reconstruction, mobility is limited, and abnormal wear at adjacent unfused joints can develop [9,10]. Simple trapezium excision avoids the problems associated with fusion, as well as the now well-understood complications of material wear and instability associated with implant arthroplasty; but weakness, instability, and proximal metacarpal migration have historically compromised long-term functional results in the absence of ligament reconstruction [11,12]. Even the addition of fascial or tendon interposition by Froimson in 1970 [13], in an effort to improve grip strength and reduce metacarpal shortening, failed to improve long-term results. This is not surprising considering the background provided earlier regarding normal TM anatomy and mechanics.

Even so, simple trapezium excision in conjunction with temporary distraction and pinning has gained recent popularity—the so-called "hematoma-distraction arthroplasty"—but long-term follow-up has not yet been reported, and the potential for a decline in pinch strength with time seems inevitable, at least in higher-demand thumbs [14]. Elsewhere in this issue, Mahoney and Meals describe a 30-minute operation time for trapeziectomy alone, but addition of a ligament reconstruction adds little time if the technique described herein is followed.

To the extent that the literature can be used to identify what is the most common treatment for basal joint arthritis today, clearly the LRTI arthroplasty procedure prevails as most popular [15–17]; however, other "suspensionplasty" procedures appear to be successful as well—emphasizing the importance of common principles:

- Trapezium excision
- Metacarpal suspension

Although tissue interposition appears to promote the repopulation of the arthroplasty space with denser, less "fatty" scar tissue, thus theoretically providing a more effective "secondary restraint" to proximal metacarpal migration over time [18], Gerwin and colleagues [19] showed that tissue interposition probably does not matter, at least in the short term. Furthermore, there does not appear to be a correlation between some degree of subsidence and outcome, unless scaphometacarpal impingement occurs—which is more likely when no ligament reconstruction has been performed [20].

In that light, in addition to the LRTI procedure, for which the entire width of the flexor carpi radialis (FCR) tendon is commonly used without morbidity [16] and a bony channel is made through the metacarpal base, Thompson [21] has been credited with describing use of a slip of the APL tendon using tunnels through both thumb and index metacarpal bases. Others have avoided the use of any bony tunnel, simply weaving a slip of abductor pollicis longus (APL) around the FCR, and sewing it back dorsally to itself or periosteum [22,23]. Weilby [24] originated this variant by describing a suspension weave of one half of the FCR looped around the AP. The world's literature uniformly describes favorable outcome following such suspensionplasties, characterized by excellent pain relief and significant improvement in strength. Patients have been very satisfied with the performance of their thumbs during activities that involve forceful grasp and lateral pinch.

The author believes that the value of "suspensionplasty" is probably more related to the provision of a volar "sling" or restraint against cantilever bending forces, which would result, in its absence, in longitudinal collapse and weakened grip, long-term. The literature certainly suggests this inevitability.

Surgical indications

Indications for surgical treatment of basal joint disease of the thumb include pain, deformity, or weakness that interferes with daily function and is unresponsive to nonoperative measures. Historically, radiographic staging has facilitated a "stage-dependent" treatment approach in which ligament reconstruction was recommended for stage 1 disease, hemitrapeziectomy, TM fusion, or implant arthroplasty for stages 2 and 3 (TM arthritis only), and complete trapezium excision with or without ligament reconstruction for stage 4 disease (pantrapezial arthritis) (Fig. 1).

Currently, for the most part, stage 1 disease continues to deserve special mention, and is typically treated with either ligament reconstruction or metacarpal extension osteotomy. Treatment of all remaining stages can be lumped together—few surgeons today preferentially perform a hemitrapeziectomy for stages 2 and 3 because of the technical ease and the benefit of improved restoration of the breadth of the thumb-index web when complete trapeziectomy is performed. Obviously pantrapezial involvement contraindicates procedures such as TM arthrodesis or hemitrapeziectomy alone.

The author specifically describes the technique of APL suspensionplasty in this article, because he relies exclusively on this procedure for treatment of all stages of basal joint disease beyond stage 1.

Abductor pollicis longus suspensionplasty: surgical technique

Incision and deep dissection

A 6-cm curvilinear incision is made from 2 finger breadths proximal to the radial styloid process, to 1 cm distal to the base of the metacarpal (Fig. 2A). The radial artery is exposed and retracted, as are branches of the radial sensory nerve. The first extensor compartment retinaculum is released, as would be performed for De-Quervain's disease, leaving the volar attachment intact. At the myotendinous junction of the APL, the ulnarmost slip of APL is released, and freed to the level of its insertion at the metacarpal base (Fig. 2B).

The EPL and APL tendons are exposed—in between is the capsule of the TM joint. Capsulotomy is performed and the trapezium is resected after cutting it partially into four fragments with a saw, and infracting it with an osteotome (Fig. 2C). The base of the thumb metacarpal is not squared off—not resecting a small sliver from the metacarpal base may help to preserve the intermetacarpal ligament.

The FCR tendon is visualized in the base of the arthroplasty space. With traction on the index and long fingers, the scapho-trapezoidal joint is inspected, and if arthritic, a resection of the proximal trapezoid is performed [17].

Creation of the abductor pollicis longus suspensionplasty

The APL slip is poked through the capsule to within the arthroplasty space, and using a right-angle clamp, passed through a slit in the FCR tendon (Fig. 2D,E). The thumb is positioned so that it rests on the index finger in the fisted position—distracted so that the metacarpal base is at the level of the index carpometacarpal (CMC) joint. A Kirschner wire is not placed. The APL slip is pulled taut, and a 3-0 vicryl suture is placed between APL slip at the level of the metacarpal base, and the extensor pollicis brevis (EPB) tendon (radially) and the tissue deep to the extensor pollicis longus (EPL) tendon (ulnarly).

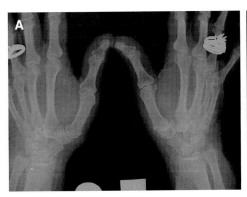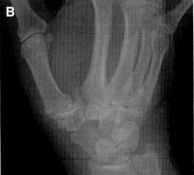

Fig. 1. (*A*) Preoperative PA stress radiograph of the right thumb, and (*B*) lateral radiograph.

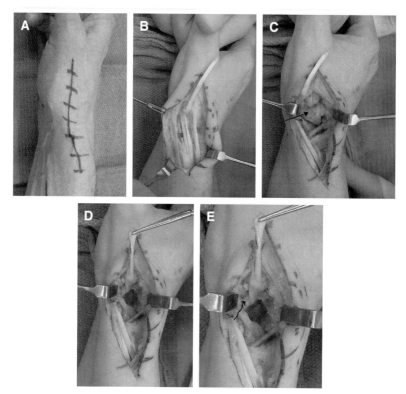

Fig. 2. APL suspensionplasty technique (*A*) Skin incision. (*B*) Distally based slip of APL. (*C*) Trapezium excision (black arrow identifies the trapezium). (*D*) Passed through/around FCR. (*E*) Magnified view (black arrow identifies the FCR tendon).

Capsular closure and rehabilitation

The capsule is closed and a thumb spica splint is placed for 10 days. At that visit a thumb spica cast is placed for 3 weeks. At approximately 4 weeks after surgery, a forearm-based thumb-spica splint is made and range-of-motion exercises begin. Opposition across the palm is avoided until 2 months after surgery, but thenar isometrics begin as soon as comfort allows. Pinch and grip strengthening generally begins around 6 to 8 weeks after surgery, and most patients are weaned from their splint by 10 weeks.

Clinical outcomes

The author's evaluation of outcomes following the APL suspensionplasty has revealed a satisfaction rate and functional return equivalent to that witnessed following the LRTI procedure in countless patients. My therapists tell me that they see no difference between the LRTI and the APL technique. Evaluation of 23 thumbs in 22 patients at a minimum of 1 year after surgery shows that grip

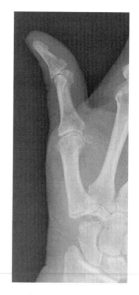

Fig. 3. Postoperative lateral radiograph shows arthroplasty space 1 year following surgery.

and key pinch strengths were 82% and 77%, respectively, compared with the opposite side (Fig. 3). Proximal migration of the metacarpal averaged 50% of the preoperative trapezial height. Experience and the literature show that modest proximal migration does not correlate with outcome [20].

In summary, APL suspensionplasty is a simple yet effective treatment alternative for basal joint arthritis. The use of a suspensionplasty technique acknowledges our current understanding of forces involved during pinch and grip, as well as the role of normal ligamentous anatomy.

References

[1] Tomaino MM. Ligament reconstruction tendon interposition arthroplasty for basal joint arthritis. Hand Clin 2001;17:207–21.

[2] Cooney WP, Chao EYS. Biomechanical analysis of static forces in the thumb during hand function. J Bone Joint Surg [Am] 1977;59:27–36.

[3] Imaeda T, An KN, Cooney WP, et al. Anatomy of trapeziometacarpal ligaments. J Hand Surg [Am] 1993;18:226–31.

[4] Bettinger P, Lindschied, Berger R, et al. An anatomic study of the stabilizing ligaments of the trapezium and trapeziometacarpal joint. J Hand Surg [Am] 1999;24:786–98.

[5] Davis TRC, Brady O, Barton NJ, et al. Trapeziectomy alone, with tendon interposition or with ligament reconstruction? J Hand Surg [Br] 1997;22:689–94.

[6] Pellegrini VD. Pathomechanics of the thumb trapeziometacarpal joint. Hand Clin 2001;17:175–84.

[7] Pellegrini VD, Olcott CW, Hollenberg G. Contact patterns in the trapeziometacarpal joint: the role of the palmar beak ligament. J Hand Surg [Am] 1993; 18:238–44.

[8] Doerschuk SH, Hicks DG, Chinchilli VM, et al. Histopathology of the palmar beak ligament in trapeziometacarpal osteoarthritis. J Hand Surg [Am] 1999;24:496–504.

[9] Bamberger HB, Stern PJ, Kiefhaber TR, et al. Trapeziometacarpal joint arthrodesis: a functional evaluation. J Hand Surg [Am] 1992;17:605–11.

[10] Hartigan BJ, Stern PJ, Kiefhaber TR. Thumb carpometacarpal osteoarthritis: arthrodesis compared with ligament reconstruction and tendon interposition. J Bone Joint Surg [Am] 2001;83:1470–8.

[11] Gervis WH. A review of excision of the trapezium for osteoarthritis of the trapezio-metacarpal joint after twenty-five years. J Bone Joint Surg [Br] 1973;55:56–7.

[12] Dell PC, Brushart TM, Smith RJ. Treatment of trapeziometacarpal arthritis: results of resection arthroplasty. J Hand Surg [Am] 1978;3:243–9.

[13] Froimson AI. Tendon arthroplasty of the trapeziometacarpal joint. Clin Orthop Rel Res 1970;70: 191–9.

[14] Kuhns CA, Emerson ET, Meals RA. Hematoma and distraction arthroplasty for thumb basal joint osteoarthritis: a prospective, single-surgeon study including outcomes measures. J Hand Surg [Am] 2003;28:381–9.

[15] Tomaino MM, Pellegrini VD, Burton RI. Arthroplasty of the basal joint of the thumb. Long-term follow up after ligament reconstruction with tendon interposition. J Bone Joint Surg [Am] 1995;77: 346–55.

[16] Tomaino MM, Coleman K. Use of the entire width of the flexor carpi radialis tendon for the LRTI arthroplasty does not impair wrist function. Am J Orthop 2000;29:283–4.

[17] Tomaino MM, Vogt M, Weiser R. Scaphotrapezoid arthritis. Prevalence in thumbs undergoing trapezium excision arthroplasty and efficacy of proximal trapezoid excision. J Hand Surg [Am] 1999;24: 1220–4.

[18] Schmidt CC, McCarthy DM, Arnoczky SP, et al. Basal joint arthroplasty using an allograft tendon interposition versus no interposition: a radiographic, vascular, and histologic study. J Hand Surg [Am] 2000;25:447–57.

[19] Gerwin M, Griffith A, Weiland AJ, et al. Ligament reconstruction basal joint arthroplasty without tendon interposition. Clin Orthop 1997;342: 42–5.

[20] Kriegs-Au G, Petje G, Fojtl E, et al. Ligament reconstruction with or without tendon interposition to treat primary thumb carpometacarpal osteoarthritis. J Bone Joint Surg [Am] 2004;86:209–18.

[21] Thompson JS. Complications and salvage of trapeziometacarpal arthritis. AAOS Instructional Course Lectures 1989;38:3–13.

[22] Sigfusson R, Lundborg G. Abductor pollicis longus tendon arthroplasty for treatment of arthrosis in the first carpometacarpal joint. Scand J Plast Reconstr Surg Hand Surg 1991;25:73–7.

[23] Nylen S, Juhlin LJ, Lugnegard H. Weilby tendon interposition arthroplasty for osteoarthritis of the trapezial joints. J Hand Surg [Br] 1987;12:68–72.

[24] Weilby A. Tendon interposition arthroplasty of the first carpo-metacarpal joint. J Hand Surg [Br] 1988;13:421–5.

ELSEVIER
SAUNDERS

Hand Clin 22 (2006) 177–182

Rheumatoid Arthritis: Silicone Metacarpophalangeal Joint Arthroplasty Indications, Technique, and Outcomes

Charles A. Goldfarb, MD[a],*, Thomas T. Dovan, MD[b]

[a]Department of Orthopaedic Surgery, Washington University School of Medicine at Barnes-Jewish Hospital,
660 South Euclid Avenue, Campus Box 8233, St. Louis, MO 63110, USA
[b]Orthopaedic & Sports Medicine Center, 301 West 6th Street SW, Rome, GA 30165, USA

Rheumatoid arthritis (RA) is a synovial-based disease that commonly affects the metacarpophalangeal (MCP) joints of the hand. The classic, end-stage MCP joint deformity is flexion and ulnar deviation with subluxation or dislocation. Although the etiology of the deformity is not entirely understood, a proliferative synovitis causes destruction of the articular surfaces and a loss of the supporting structures of the joint. Other contributing factors include exaggeration of the ulnar shift of the long flexors, the ulnar pull of the intrinsic musculature, and the bony anatomy of the MCP joint articulation. The disease is not isolated to the MCP joints; the classic wrist collapse leads to radial deviation of the metacarpals, further exaggerating the deforming forces at the MCP joint. Volar subluxation or dislocation may be the result of unopposed flexor tendon forces on the attenuated capsular structures [1–3].

Traditionally, it has been taught that surgical intervention should be considered when MCP deformity severely limits function. This was based on reports of objective improvements in MCP joint extension and some overall improvement in MCP joint motion [4–14]. The recent use of patient-centered outcomes measures has demonstrated that function is subjectively improved by the arthroplasty; additionally, the improvements in appearance and pain control are highly valued

by patients [15,16]. It is important to emphasize the evidence-based considerations to the patients and stress to them that the decision for surgery is a patient-centered decision.

Operative intervention at the MCP joints must be preceded by the correction of more proximal joint alignment problems. If the wrist is radially deviated, a partial or complete wrist fusion should be considered to axially align the wrist joint; the authors' preference, when possible, is the radiolunate fusion. Soft-tissue procedures and synovectomy are not sufficient when the wrist is malaligned. Failure to correct a radially-deviated wrist before treatment of the MCP joints will likely lead to a failure of the operative treatment at the MCP joints.

Two classes of operative intervention exist for the MCP joint: soft tissue stabilization/realignment and arthroplasty [5,9,17]. Early disease at the MCP joint can be treated with MCP joint synovectomy [18,19], a procedure that may delay progression of disease. Additionally, tendon subluxation without joint subluxation or dislocation can be treated with extensor tendon realignment. Once there is radiographic evidence of joint destruction, joint subluxation or dislocation, significant ulnar drift, and contracted intrinsic and extrinsic muscles with associated stiff interphalangeal joints, soft-tissue procedures will not suffice [17]. MCP arthroplasty in these patients who have advanced disease should be considered for pain, functional limitations, or severe aesthetic deformity.

There is a subset of patients who have joint subluxation, ulnar drift, and advanced radiographic

* Corresponding author.
  E-mail address: goldfarbc@wustl.edu
(C.A. Goldfarb).

changes who remain pain free and demonstrate good hand function. These patients are best treated with night splints and observation. Surgery will not increase their function and may weaken their grip strength [20].

Metacarpophalangeal joint arthroplasty

MCP joint arthroplasty is designed to relieve pain, restore function, and correct deformity to provide an aesthetic improvement to the hand. Many prosthetic designs have been introduced over the last 40 years, and these may be grouped into one of three basic designs: the hinged prosthesis, the flexible prosthesis, and the third-generation prosthesis. The early, hinged designs included the Brannon and Klein, Flatt, Griffith-Nicolle, Schetrumpf, Schultz, Steffee, St. Beorg-Buchholtz, KY alumina, and the Minami alumina prostheses [21]. The hinged prosthesis is no longer regularly used because of its high failure rate.

The Swanson silicone implant has been used for more than 40 years and remains the gold standard for MCP arthroplasty in RA. The silicone MCP joint arthroplasty is based on Swanson's theory of joint encapsulation; this suggests that the silicone implant serves as a joint spacer, allowing the formation of scar tissue to provide joint stability [17]. The initiation of early motion promotes the development of a functionally adapted fibrous capsule during this process [22]. Additional fixation and bony ingrowth are not needed, because the implant becomes stable through the encapsulation process. In fact, rigid fixation is contraindicated—joint pistoning may increase the life of the implant because of broader implant force dispersion with joint motion. By contrast, newer preflexed box designs enable more joint flexion at the hinge.

Although Swanson implants have been effective, several shortcomings exist. First, there is high implant fracture rate of up to 63% at long-term follow-up [7]. Although the encapsulation theory suggests that implant integrity is not crucial after the immediate postoperative period [17], implant fracture has been correlated with recurrent ulnar drift and poor functional outcome [7]. When silicone implants were first developed for RA MCP disease, life expectancy was limited. The implant needed only to "outlive" the patient; however, the disease-modifying, antirheumatic drugs (DMARDS) have altered this concept. First, fewer patients develop fixed deformities at the MCP joint secondary to the early institution of the medications. Second, those patients who do come to surgery are typically under better medical control and can be expected to live for a longer duration. Implant durability is now more of a concern in the provision of a long-term solution at the MCP joint.

Secondary to the limitations and the need for implants in a younger, more active population, surface replacement prosthesis were developed. These third-generation implants recreate joint anatomy and include the Kessler, Hagert, Lunborg, and Beckenbaugh (pyrolytic carbon) prostheses. The pyrolytic carbon implant has received the most attention; the physical and mechanical properties of this isotropic material fall between those of graphite and diamond. Pyrolytic carbon MCP implants have gained in popularity, given their mechanical properties and low wear rates. This implant is an articulating, unconstrained design with a hemispherical head and grooved, offset stems. A long-term study [23] reporting a minimum 10-year follow-up shows promising results with 5- and 10-year survival rates at 82% and 81%, respectively; however, patients treated in this series had little "preoperative" deformity, subluxation, or dislocation of the MP joint. Patients who had dislocation and shortening of greater than 1 cm and patients who had advanced cortical bone loss were not treated with pyrolytic carbon implants [23]. The primary concern with these implants is their ability to resist flexion and ulnar deviation forces.

Surgical technique

A transverse incision is made between the metacarpal necks and the MCP joints, with care taken to preserve the dorsal veins. The extensor hood is exposed; the radial portion of the hood is stretched and the extensor tendons are typically dislocated between the metacarpal heads. A longitudinal incision parallel to the tendon is made on its ulnar side through the sagittal band. The tendon is mobilized with scissor dissection as necessary, and it is retracted radially to expose the dorsal joint capsule. A longitudinal incision and a subperiosteal exposure of the metacarpal neck are performed. A complete synovectomy is performed. The radial collateral ligament is tagged with a nonabsorbable 3'0 suture for later repair, and then both the radial and ulnar collateral ligaments are released from the metacarpal. The metacarpal head is excised with an oscillating saw at the level of the metaphyseal flare, with Hohman retractors used for protection. The soft tissues about the base of the proximal phalanx are released sharply; specifically, the dorsal and ulnar tissues and the volar plate are incised. The radial attachments are maintained. Once the release has been performed, the proximal phalanx should be mobile enough to allow it to be displaced dorsal to the metacarpal. If the ulnar intrinsic muscles are tight, the tendons may be withdrawn into the wound and divided.

The metacarpal is prepared first; a canal finder is used to identify the medullary canal, and sequential awls will enlarge the canal. A side-cutting burr (to avoid penetration of the cortex) may be used to enlarge the canal. When preparing the proximal phalanx, the base is not resected. A starting hole is created with a burr or an awl, and then appropriate-sized reamers are used. Trials are used and the largest implant possible should be implanted. If impingement between the metacarpal or proximal phalanx and the implant is present with the joint extended, additional bone should be resected or further soft tissue releases performed. The ring finger usually requires the smallest implant. The radial collateral ligament may be repaired through a drill hole to the metacarpal; this may be performed for all joints or only in the index finger. The implant is then placed (the authors do not use grommets). During closure, the radial portion of the extensor hood is reefed to help realign the extensor tendon or to bring it slightly to the radial side of the center of the joint [17]. The tourniquet is deflated before closure for hemostasis, and a silastic drain is maintained for passive drainage for 24 to 48 hours.

Postoperative care

A bulky hand dressing is applied for 4 to 7 days. When the initial postoperative dressing is removed, the patient is fitted with a dynamic outrigger orthoplast splint to maintain MCP extension and slight radial deviation [24]. Early active range of motion is begun under the supervision of a hand therapist for a 6- to 8-week program. The patient is instructed on joint protection procedures to avoid excessive ulnar-deviation forces. At 6 weeks, the dynamic splint is discontinued and the patient wears a nighttime extension splint for up to 4 months, depending on the amount of extensor lag at the MP joints.

Outcomes

The outcomes literature concerning MCP arthroplasty is replete with retrospective reports with limited clinical and radiographic data. These reports, of varying follow-up duration, have typically included clinical information on finger alignment and joint range of motion with radiographic data including implant fracture rate. The reports (Table 1) have provided valuable data that have, on most issues, been homogeneous. At less than 10-year follow-up, improved function was noted in 60% to 75% of patients, improved appearance was noted in 42% to 82% of patients, and pain was present in up to 50% of patients [4–14]. These data have been used by most investigators to justify silicone implant arthroplasty but, for at least one set of investigators, these data have led to a discontinuance of the procedure [12].

The specific data from the most recent long-term follow-up investigation provide a review of

Table 1
Intermediate and long-term outcomes of MCP arthroplasty

Investigation	# joints	F/U (years)	Active MCP ROM	Implant fracture
Mannerfelt et al [10]	144	2.5	40	4/144 (3%)
Beckenbaugh et al [4]	186	2.8	38	31/186 (16%)
Blair et al [6]	115	4.5	43	24/115 (21%)
Bieber et al [5]	210	5	39	0/210 (0%)
Maurer et al [11]	137	8.4	39	
Kirshenbaum et al [9]	144	8.5	44	15/144 (10%)
Wilson et al [3]	185	9.5	29	
Olsen et al [12]	60	7	30	13/60 (22%)
Hansraj et al [8]	170	5.2	27	12/170 (7%)
Schmidt et al [13]	102	10.1	35	28/102 (28%)
Goldfarb and Stern [7]	208	14.2	36	134/208 (63%)

Abbreviations: F/U, Followup; ROM, range of motion.

this information [7]. In this investigation, 36 patients who had 208 MCP joint arthroplasties were evaluated at an average of 14 years after surgery. Active MCP motion improved after surgery, and the MCP joints were held in a more extended, and thus more functional, posture. The preoperative MCP joint arc of motion was 57° to 87° (arc 30°), the immediate postoperative arc of motion was 11° to 57° (arc 46°), and the final arc of motion was 23° to 59° (arc 36°). Although the total motion improved only 6°, the arc of motion was moved approximately 30° toward extension. MCP joint axial alignment was not maintained at final follow-up. Preoperative ulnar deviation averaged 26°, immediate postoperative values were less than 5°, and final follow-up, ulnar deviation averaged 16°. Those patients who had implant fractures had a greater degree of ulnar drift recurrence: 10° versus 20° of ulnar drift. The implant fracture rate was 63%, and another 22% of the implants were deformed. The Sutter implants were fractured in 52% of joints compared with 67% in the Swanson implants. Table 1 summarizes these reports.

Although these outcome reports provide valuable information, the literature has been deficient in several areas. The lack of prospective, randomized studies using validated outcomes instruments that target the outcome measures most important to RA patients has hindered our ability to truly understand patient outcome. These deficits are, at least in part, responsible for the significant difference between rheumatologists and hand surgeons in their opinions of the effectiveness of MCP joint arthroplasty and hand surgery in general for RA patients. A mailed survey of 500 hand surgeons and 500 rheumatologists was used to assess current practice and beliefs regarding RA and hand surgery [25,26]. The data demonstrated a marked disparity in opinions between the two groups. Seventy percent of the rheumatologists felt that the hand surgeons had deficient knowledge of medical treatment, and 74% of the surgeons felt the rheumatologists' knowledge of surgical options was deficient. The study noted that there was minimal cross-training between the two groups. Age of the survey responders and other biographical information did not significantly affect the results.

The two groups had a dramatic difference of opinion concerning the indications for and opinions of outcomes of hand surgery in RA. Opinions were different for all procedures, including extensor synovectomy, distal ulna resection, wrist fusion, small joint synovectomy, and small-joint

soft-tissue correction. The findings for MCP arthroplasty highlight the differences in opinions between hand surgeons to rheumatologists. Eighty two percent of hand surgeons felt that MCP arthroplasty improves function, compared with 34% of rheumatologists; 95% of hand surgeons felt that MCP arthroplasty improves hand aesthetics, compared with 67% of rheumatologists; and 33% of hand surgeons felt that surgery improves strength, compared with 24% of rheumatologists. Training and interpretation of the data in the literature may explain the difference in these opinions.

Recent reports have added significant new information toward our understanding of MCP arthroplasty. Mandl and colleagues [16] evaluated the outcome of 26 patients (160 joints) at an average 5.5 years, based on the subjective assessment of pain, appearance, work, activities of daily living, and satisfaction with function. An objective examination was performed on 18 of the patients. This report found that postoperative patient satisfaction was most correlated with hand appearance. Pain and, to a lesser degree subjective assessment of function, were also correlated with satisfaction. Objective measures such as strength and range of motion were only minimally correlated with patient satisfaction [16]. This investigation emphasizes that patient determinants of success must be used in assessing surgical outcome.

Chung and coworkers [15] have reported the early outcome of MCP arthroplasty in a prospective assessment at 6 months and 12 months using a functional assessment, the Michigan Hand Questionnaire (MHQ), and the Arthritis Impact Measurement Scale (AIMS). At 1 year, there was no significant difference in grip strength, the Jebsen test, or MCP joint range of motion (although improved by an average of 13°). Ulnar drift was significantly improved. Most notably, MHQ scores were significantly improved in all areas (function, activities of daily living [ADL], pain, aesthetics, and satisfaction) except work. This investigation also emphasizes the importance of patient-centered determinants of outcome; patients were clearly subjectively improved at 1 year after surgery [15]. Both this study and the Mandl investigation are optimistic about the outcomes of MCP arthroplasty if specific, patient-centered measures are used.

The Swanson silicone MCP arthroplasty was introduced in 1962, and the Sutter implant was introduced in 1987 [17]. The Sutter implant (currently marketed under the name Avanta) is similar to the Swanson implant but has a different geometric design, with a center of flexion palmar to the longitudinal axis. It was thought that these changes would allow more flexion and better postoperative function. The new implant had been widely adopted until Bass and Stern [27] reported a markedly higher fracture rate (45% at 3 years) compared with the Swanson implant at short-term assessment. The study authors concluded that they could not, therefore, recommend the use of the implant. Interestingly, a recent investigation with 14 year follow-up [7] found similar fracture rates when comparing the Swanson with the Sutter implant (58% and 52%, respectively).

Recently, a prospective, randomized assessment of the two implants in 30 patients was reported with 2-year follow-up. Similar to the findings in the Chung [15] and the Mandl [16] investigations, objective measures of grip strength and hand function were unchanged. Visual analog scales demonstrated significant subjective improvements in pain, hand function, grip strength, and appearance. Flexion and ulnar deviation deformity improved in both groups to a significant degree. Although the Avanta implant group demonstrated an arc of motion 7° greater than the arc of motion in the Swanson group, this difference was not significant. The Avanta fractures rate was greater (12 fractures, 20%) than the Swanson (8 fractures, 13%) implants, but this difference did not reach statistical significance [28].

The incidence of radiographic osteolysis after MCP arthroplasty was evaluated with a prospective, randomized evaluation of the Swanson and the Sutter prostheses [29]. Seventy-five Swanson implants and 99 Sutter implants were radiographically evaluated at 58 months postoperatively. The osteolytic changes were graded from I to IV. The Sutter group had a significantly increased rate of osteolysis when compared with the Swanson implants. The study authors suggested use of implant arthroplasty only when other surgical alternatives are not available. They also suggested that, even at short-term follow-up, the use of the Sutter implant was questionable. The affect of silicone arthroplasty on the adjacent bone has been noted in other investigations as well. Metacarpal and proximal phalanx shortening, osteolysis around the implants, and subsidence were all noted to be problematic at long-term follow-up. Additionally, certain patients were more severely affected with marked shortening of the metacarpals in 6 of 18 hands [7].

The silicone implant arthroplasty can be an effective treatment option for in RA with severe disease at the MCP joints. Ideally, medical management is used to bring the systemic disease under control before arthroplasty. Although objective improvement after MCP arthroplasty may be limited, the use of patient-centered data has confirmed the utility of the procedure. MCP joint arthroplasty is an effective treatment option from a patient-centered perspective, in that it can improve appearance, pain, and function. The use of DMARDS has made the surgical treatment of RA less common; however, in those patients that undergo MCP arthroplasty, implants are needed that will provide long-term stability with minimal bone reaction.

References

[1] Shapiro JS. Ulnar drift. Report of a related finding. Acta Orthop Scand 1968;39(3):346–53.

[2] Shapiro JS. A new factor in the etiology of ulnar drift. Clin Orthop Relat Res 1970;68:32–43.

[3] Wilson RL, Carlblom ER. The rheumatoid metacarpophalangeal joint. Hand Clin 1989;5(2):223–37.

[4] Beckenbaugh RD, Dobyns JH, Linscheid RL, et al. Review and analysis of silicone-rubber metacarpophalangeal implants. J Bone Joint Surg Am 1976; 58(4):483–7.

[5] Bieber EJ, Weiland AJ, Volenec-Dowling S. Silicone-rubber implant arthroplasty of the metacarpophalangeal joints for rheumatoid arthritis. J Bone Joint Surg Am 1986;68(2):206–9.

[6] Blair WF, Shurr DG, Buckwalter JA. Metacarpophalangeal joint implant arthroplasty with a Silastic spacer. J Bone Joint Surg Am 1984;66(3):365–70.

[7] Goldfarb CA, Stern PJ. Metacarpophalangeal joint arthroplasty in rheumatoid arthritis. A long-term assessment. J Bone Joint Surg Am 2003;85-A(10): 1869–78.

[8] Hansraj KK, Ashworth CR, Ebramzadeh E, et al. Swanson metacarpophalangeal joint arthroplasty in patients with rheumatoid arthritis. Clin Orthop Relat Res 1997;342:11–5.

[9] Kirschenbaum D, Schneider LH, Adams DC, et al. Arthroplasty of the metacarpophalangeal joints with use of silicone-rubber implants in patients who have rheumatoid arthritis. Long-term results. J Bone Joint Surg Am 1993;75(1):3–12.

[10] Mannerfelt L, Andersson K. Silastic arthroplasty of the metacarpophalangeal joints in rheumatoid arthritis. J Bone Joint Surg Am 1975;57(4):484–9.

[11] Maurer RJ, Ranawat CS, McCormack RR, et al. Long-term follow-up of the Swanson MP arthroplasty for rheumatoid arthritis. Proceedings of ASSH [abstract]. J Hand Surg [Am] 1990;15:810–1.

[12] Olsen I, Gebuhr P, Sonne-Holm S. Silastic arthroplasty in rheumatoid MCP-joints. 60 joints followed for 7 years. Acta Orthop Scand 1994;65(4):430–1.

[13] Schmidt K, Willburger RE, Miehlke RK, et al. Ten-year follow-up of silicone arthroplasty of the metacarpophalangeal joints in rheumatoid hands. Scand J Plast Reconstr Surg Hand Surg 1999;33(4):433–8.

[14] Wilson YG, Sykes PJ, Niranjan NS. Long-term follow-up of Swanson's silastic arthroplasty of the metacarpophalangeal joints in rheumatoid arthritis. J Hand Surg [Br] 1993;18(1):81–91.

[15] Chung KC, Kotsis SV, Kim HM. A prospective outcomes study of Swanson metacarpophalangeal joint arthroplasty for the rheumatoid hand. J Hand Surg [Am] 2004;29(4):646–53.

[16] Mandl LA, Galvin DH, Bosch JP, et al. Metacarpophalangeal arthroplasty in rheumatoid arthritis: what determines satisfaction with surgery? J Rheumatol 2002;29(12):2488–91.

[17] Swanson AB. Flexible implant arthroplasty for arthritic finger joints: rationale, technique, and results of treatment. J Bone Joint Surg Am 1972;54(3):435–55.

[18] Cleland LG, Treganza R, Dobson P. Arthroscopic synovectomy: a prospective study. J Rheumatol 1986;13(5):907–10.

[19] Edstrom B, Lugnegard H, Syk B. Late synovectomy of the hand in rheumatoid arthritis. Scand J Rheumatol 1976;5(3):184–90.

[20] Feldon P, Terrono Al, Nalebuff EA, et al. Rheumatoid arthritis and other connective tissues diseases. In: Green DP, editor. Operative hand surgery, 4th edition: New York: Churchill Livingstone; 1999. p. 1651–739.

[21] Beevers DJ, Seedhom BB. Metacarpophalangeal joint prostheses. A review of the clinical results of past and current designs. J Hand Surg [Br] 1995; 20(2):125–36.

[22] Swanson AB. Finger joint replacement by silicone rubber implants and the concept of implant fixation by encapsulation. Ann Rheum Dis 1969;28: (5)(Suppl):47–55.

[23] Cook SD, Beckenbaugh RD, Redondo J, et al. Long-term follow-up of pyrolytic carbon metacarpophalangeal implants. J Bone Joint Surg Am 1999;81(5):635–48.

[24] Thomsen NO, Boeckstyns ME, Leth-Espensen P. Value of dynamic splinting after replacement of the metacarpophalangeal joint in patients with rheumatoid arthritis. Scand J Plast Reconstr Surg Hand Surg 2003;37(2):113–6.

[25] Alderman AK, Chung KC, Kim HM, et al. Effectiveness of rheumatoid hand surgery: contrasting perceptions of hand surgeons and rheumatologists. J Hand Surg [Am] 2003;28(1):3–11 [discussion: 12–3].

[26] Alderman AK, Ubel PA, Kim HM, et al. Surgical management of the rheumatoid hand: consensus and controversy among rheumatologists and hand surgeons. J Rheumatol 2003;30(7):1464–72.

[27] Bass RL, Stern PJ, Nairus JG. High implant fracture incidence with Sutter silicone metacarpophalangeal joint arthroplasty. J Hand Surg [Am] 1996;21(5): 813–8.

[28] Moller K, Sollerman C, Geijer M, et al. Avanta versus Swanson silicone implants in the MCP joint–a prospective, randomized comparison of 30 patients followed for 2 years. J Hand Surg [Br] 2005;30(1):8–13.

[29] Parkkila TJ, Belt EA, Hakala M, et al. Grading of radiographic osteolytic changes after silastic metacarpophalangeal arthroplasty and a prospective trial of osteolysis following use of Swanson and Sutter prostheses. J Hand Surg [Br] 2005;30(4): 382–7.

ELSEVIER
SAUNDERS

Hand Clin 22 (2006) 183–193

HAND
CLINICS

Nonrheumatoid Metacarpophalangeal Joint Arthritis. Unconstrained Pyrolytic Carbon Implants: Indications, Technique, and Outcomes

Wendy Parker, MD, PhD[a], Steven L. Moran, MD[a,b,*],
Kirsten B. Hormel, RN[a], Marco Rizzo, MD[a],
Robert D. Beckenbaugh, MD[a]

[a]Department of Orthopedic Surgery, Mayo Clinic College of Medicine,
200 First Street SW, Rochester, MN 55905, USA
[b]Division of Plastic Surgery, Mayo Clinic College of Medicine, 200 First Street SW, Rochester, MN 55905, USA

Beginning with the introduction of soft-tissue arthroplasty, there have been multiple attempts to create an ideal and long lasting metacarpophalangeal (MP) joint arthroplasty; design types have included hinged [1–5], semiconstrained [6–8], and unconstrained instrumentation [9–13]. Although many of these implants have been associated with early pain relief, they have also resulted in progressive ulnar drift, bone loss, and decreasing hand function over time [6,7,12,13]. Pyrolytic carbon implants offer advantages over previously used polyethylene and metal implants. Pyrolytic carbon has an elastic modulus that is similar to cortical bone, which aids in dampening stresses at the bone prosthetic interface and enhances biological fixation. In addition, pyrolytic carbon has been found to have excellent long-term biological compatibility [14,15].

The predominant implant in use today remains the silicone-elastomer constrained implant [16]. Silicone implants, although providing pain relief and improving cosmesis, have also been associated with progressive bone destruction, fracture, and deterioration in hand function [17–19].

Mechanical failure rates are high, with as many as 82% of implants fracturing after 5 years [12,13,20,21].

The majority of MP joint arthroplasties are performed for rheumatoid arthritis; however osteoarthritis (OA) of the MP joint is not uncommon and can also render the MP joint nonfunctional. OA of the MP joint primarily affects the index and long fingers. Application of silastic implants in this setting, where surrounding hand function is strong, can result in early failure, displacement, and lateral instability. Unconstrained implants may provide benefits in this situation when the soft-tissue constraints remain intact in general. With the development of unconstrained MP joint replacement, salvage of this joint may be performed reliably in patients who have primary OA and post-traumatic arthritis (TA) of the MP joint.

Biomechanical considerations and potential benefits of unconstrained implants

Unlike the ginglymoid IP joint, which functions like a sloppy hinge joint, the condyloid MP joint is diarthrodial, with three degrees of freedom, allowing for flexion-extension, abduction-adduction, and some rotation [12,22]. Most prehension grips require that the digits extend and abduct at the MP joint. In the last 30° of flexion, the collateral ligaments become more taut and

* Corresponding author. Division of Plastic Surgery, Mayo Clinic College of Medicine, 200 First Street SW, Rochester, MN 55905.
E-mail address: moran.steven@mayo.edu (S.L. Moran).

0749-0712/06/$ - see front matter © 2006 Elsevier Inc. All rights reserved.
doi:10.1016/j.hcl.2006.02.012

hand.theclinics.com

the condylar configuration of the joint shifts the joint contact areas laterally [23–32]. At this point the joint primarily functions as a hinge joint, with two degrees of freedom because of the constraints of the collateral ligaments [33].

In general, constrained implant designs allow for two degrees of freedom, permitting primarily flexion or extension. During the extremes of flexion and extension, hinged and constrained prostheses suffer from the inherent problem of reciprocal displacement of the joint's center of rotation. Displacement of the joint's axle during flexion and extension changes the moment arm to favor persistence of one or the other extreme of positioning [33]. Unconstrained design can allow for a virtual rather than fixed axis as its center of rotation. A virtual axis allows for a combination of rolling and sliding movements that at the extremes of motion will leave the antagonist muscles with an improved mechanical advantage for the initiation of flexion or extension [33,34].

Constrained implants often require large bony resection, resulting in compromise of the collateral ligaments. The collateral ligaments and accessory collateral ligaments help resist lateral and palmar subluxating forces [25,35–37]. If they are excised during implant placement, resistance to subluxation is significantly compromised, whereas intact collateral ligaments are capable of transmitting deforming stresses to the cortical bone. Constrained implants and cemented components transmit stress primarily to the endosteal surface, inducing cellular injury at the prosthesis-bone interface [25,37–41].

Pyrolytic carbon arthroplasty allows for preservation of the collateral ligaments and accessory collateral ligaments. Preservation of these structures helps divert subluxating and out-of-plane forces away from the prosthesis to the ligamentous insertions on the cortical surface [33,42]. Minimal joint resection also leaves a wider surface area for the dissipation and distribution of the joint's compressive loads. In addition, release or resection of the collateral and accessory collateral ligaments allows for ulnopalmar bowstringing of the flexor tendons. This results in an increase in the flexor tendon moment arm, encouraging the development of a flexion contracture and ulnar deviation of the digit [30,32,33,37,43–45].

The theoretical disadvantage of the unconstrained MP joint design is the possibility of subluxation and dislocation, particularly when the surrounding soft tissue is loose or damaged, as in cases of inflammatory arthritis

[10,23,33,39,42–44,46,47]. Unconstrained implants do require precise placement of the implant stems to ensure preservation of the rotational axis and the sagittal moment arms. In its native state, the joint is balanced because of the moment arms created by flexion and extension forces passing at fixed distances from the joint's center of rotation. Improper placement of the prosthesis or inadequate sizing of the prosthesis tends to result in improper soft-tissue balancing, which may tend to push the phalanx into flexion or extension. Dorsally displaced components can lead to a postoperative flexion deformity caused by the increase in moment arm force. Palmarly positioned components will induce extension posturing of the finger postoperatively [36,46,48–52].

Stem placement must be closely examined in the coronal plane as well. The contours of the index and long-finger metacarpal heads are asymmetric; this is of particular importance in OA, in which the index and long fingers are most commonly affected. In the joint's native state, this asymmetry favors appositional pinch by providing a larger moment arm for the radial intrinsics [23,33,47] To maintain this favorable soft-tissue balance in the index finger, the metacarpal component of the implant should be offset slightly ulnarly to compensate for the implant's symmetric contour. Radial positioning of the metacarpal component should be avoided because this will further increase the radial deviating moment arm, encouraging ulnar drift [33].

Indications

The most important factors for long-term stability of an unconstrained implant are a stable soft-tissue envelope and adequate bone stock to allow for fixation through appositional bone growth. The ideal patients for pyrolytic carbon MP joint replacement are OA and TA patients. In the majority of OA and TA patients, the soft-tissue envelope surrounding the MP joint is stable and often thickened, providing added stability following arthroplasty. In addition, the bone quality is excellent and allows for stable fixation with little room for implant subsidence.

Despite this, RA remains the most common indication for MP arthroplasty at the authors' institution. RA presents the most concerns for the surgeon with regards to soft-tissue impairment and ongoing destruction of the joint capsule, ligaments, and tendons. RA patients also present with varying degrees of osteolysis and osteoporosis. Both of these factors may lead to secondary displacement, migration, or implant subsidence. Patients who have RA and who have soft medullary bone or thin cortical bone and significant destruction or imbalance of the soft tissues should be approached with caution. If there is severe deformity with greater than 80°s of an extension lag or more than 45° of ulnar deviation, the use of standard silicone implants may be necessary. In cases of complete MP joint dislocation with proximal migration of the proximal phalanx, a pyrolytic implant should not be used [14]. Patients who fail arthroplasty because of recurrent subluxation or migration may be salvaged by revising the joint with a constrained silicone implant. Wrist stability should also be achieved before MP joint replacement, particularly in RA patients who have significant intercarpal supination, radial deviation, and ulnar translocation of the wrist. Relative contraindications for pyrolytic carbon implant placement also include loss of extensor function, inadequate dorsal soft-tissue, and evidence of recent infection.

Surgical technique

The operation is performed through a dorsal or longitudinal incision created over the MP joint (Fig. 1). If the extensor tendons are intact and not displaced ulnarly, the extensor mechanism is opened longitudinally over the joint. If the extensor tendon is subluxed, the sagittal bands are incised on the radial side of the central tendon to facilitate centralization at the completion of the case. The extensor hood is separated from the capsule, and the capsule is then incised in a longitudinal fashion.

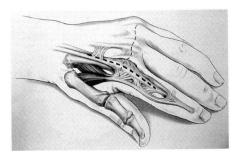

Fig. 1. The operation may be performed through a transverse or straight dorsal incision. The joint is approached through a central splitting approach if the tendon is not subluxed. (© Mayo Clinic Foundation, used with permission.)

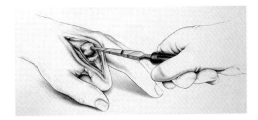

Fig. 2. A starter awl is used to identify the medullary canal. (© Mayo Clinic Foundation, used with permission.)

Excess synovium is removed in addition to any large dorsal osteophytes.

With the joint exposed, the starter awl is used to identify the medullary canal of the metacarpal (Fig. 2). The alignment and cutting guide is then placed within the medullary canal (Fig. 3). An oscillating saw is placed within the saw guide and used to start the cut dorsally to the center of the guide (Fig. 4). The angle of the cut is 27.5°. Once the osteotomy has been initiated, the guide is removed and the remaining portion of the osteotomy is completed freehand (Fig. 5).

The proximal phalanx is then prepared using the same sequence as was used for the metacarpal osteotomy (Fig. 6). The cutting guide for the proximal phalanx provides a 5° back cut (Fig. 7). During both proximal and distal osteotomies every attempt is made to preserve the collateral ligaments and as much bone length as possible.

The medullary canals of both the metacarpal and proximal phalanx are now prepared with the broaches (Fig. 8). The medullary bone is impacted; however, in cases of significantly sclerotic bone (as is the case in many patients with OA), the canal may need to be enlarged with a side-cutting burr. The canals of the metacarpal and proximal phalanx are prepared until they are able to accept the largest implant that will fit in the proximal phalanx. Intraoperative fluoroscopy is used

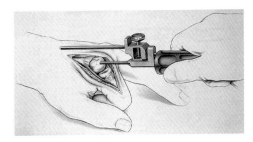

Fig. 3. An alignment guide is inserted into the metacarpal to centralize the cut for the metacarpal head. (© Mayo Clinic Foundation, used with permission.)

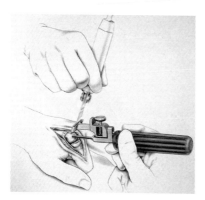

Fig. 4. The saw guide produces a 27.5° angled osteotomy of the metacarpal head. (© Mayo Clinic Foundation, used with permission.)

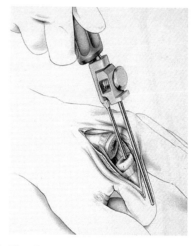

Fig. 6. The alignment guide is placed into the proximal phalanx. (© Mayo Clinic Foundation, used with permission.)

liberally throughout the case to ensure central placement of all broaches and awls within the coronal and sagittal planes. Implants should not be mismatches; this differs from proximal interphalangeal joint surface replacement arthroplasties, in which mismatching between the proximal and distal component is possible. Broaching is stopped when the sized reamers are seated just below the bone edge. Final implants tend to be slightly larger than trial components (Fig. 9). Trial implants are then placed and the joint is reduced. The MP joint should move passively through a 0° to 90° arc without significant tension (Fig. 10). In patients who have longstanding osteoarthritis or post-traumatic arthritis, when flexor contractures are present, release of the volar plate or intrinsic release and reinsertion may also be necessary to gain full extension. Ulnar release is often required in rheumatoid patients for joint rebalancing.

Trial implants are removed and permanent implants are placed. Dorsal and palmar stability are tested, and collateral ligaments are reinserted if they required resection or release during implant placement. Fluoroscopy is used to verify implant position before closure. The dorsal capsule is trimmed to allow for a snug repair over the prosthesis. The extensor mechanism is closed with radial imbrication of the hood to centralize the tendon over the MCP joint (Fig. 11). In cases of RA, the ulnar hood can be cut free of the central tendon if it is too tight to allow for imbrication. The remainder of the wound is closed in the standard fashion. The hand dressing is applied to maintain the digits in extension at the MP joint and allow for some functional flexion at the interphalangeal joints. Radiographs are taken in the postoperative

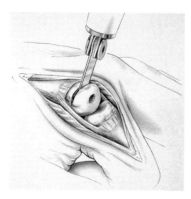

Fig 5. The angled osteotomy on the metacarpal head is completed freehand after the cut has been initiated with the saw guide. (© Mayo Clinic Foundation, used with permission.)

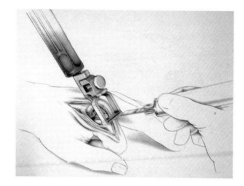

Fig. 7. The proximal phalanx saw guide is then used to create a 5° back cut. (© Mayo Clinic Foundation, used with permission.)

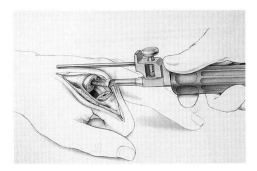

Fig. 8. Broaches are used to prepare the medullary canal. (© Mayo Clinic Foundation, used with permission.)

dressing to ensure there has been no subluxation during dressing application.

Postoperative care

Because of the unconstrained design of the implant, some soft-tissue healing must occur to provide initial stability. In the patient who has osteoarthritis, when soft-tissue stability is good, short-arc MP joint motion may be allowed as early as 4 to 7 days postoperative under careful supervision of a therapist. Motion is protected initially with dynamic and static splints (Fig. 12A,B). MP joint motion is gradually increased on a weekly basis. Light activities are allowed while the splints are being worn. In patients undergoing a single MP joint replacement, protective buddy tapping may be initiated at 1 month. Patients are weaned from the splints at 6 weeks. In the rheumatoid patient, the MP joint is immobilized in full extension for 3 to 4 weeks, with some interphalangeal motion allowed after 7 to 10 days. Early motion, as would be

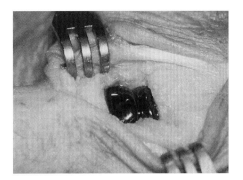

Fig. 10. Position and appearance of a reduced implant before closure.

allowed with silicone arthroplasty, should not be allowed with pyrolytic carbon implants because significant flexion may lead to instability.

Outcome study

Methods

A total of 21 MP joint arthroplasties in 19 patients were performed for OA over the past 3 years at the authors' institution. Ten of these patients were part of a prospective Food and Drug Administration (FDA)-approved study and the remaining 9 opted out of the study protocol, but were reviewed retrospectively. All patients presenting with OA of the MP joint were requested to participate in the study.

All patients completed questionnaires preoperatively, and at 6 weeks, 12 weeks, 6 months, and 1 year following surgery. The questionnaires inquired about patient age, sex, race, hand dominance, history of trauma, and previous surgical procedures performed on the involved joint. Patients were asked to give their major reason

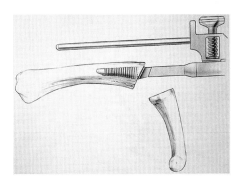

Fig. 9. An impactor broach is then fully seated in the proximal phalanx to allow press fit of the final implant; a similar procedure is performed with the metacarpal component. (© Mayo Clinic Foundation, used with permission.)

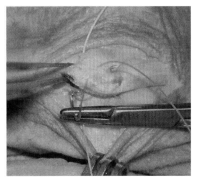

Fig. 11. Extensor mechanism is closed with radial imbrication.

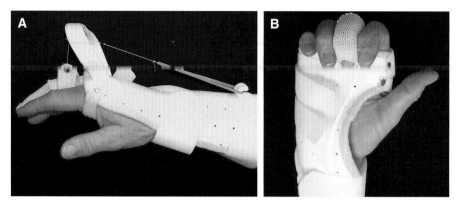

Fig. 12. (*A*) Dynamic extension splint is worn after the first postoperative visit for the first 3 to 4 weeks as multiple joints are replaced. (*B*) Modification of the splint to allow for proximal interphalangeal (PIP) flexion; static splints are worn at night.

for proceeding with surgery. They were also asked to document their employment status preoperatively and at all postoperative time points.

Patients recorded their postoperative progress using visual analog scales. Visual analog scales evaluated pain, function, and cosmesis of the finger. All findings were marked on a linear, nongraduated scale from 0 to 100. These markings were measured with a ruler to determine the percent rating of pain, the percent of normal functioning of the digit, and percent of normal appearance as subjectively determined by the patient.

Measurements of MP joint flexion, extension lag, and radial or ulnar deviation were obtained. Oppositional pinch and grip strengths were obtained for all time points apart from the 6-week postoperative period, where it was felt that over-exertion may displace the implant or cause soft-tissue injury. All data were collected using the standardized computer assisted hand measurement tools (Dexter system). Strength measurements were performed in triplicate and averaged. All data were organized on a standard excel spreadsheet and tabulated. A student *t*-test was used for all statistical comparisons.

Radiological assessment was performed preoperatively, and 1 week, 6 weeks, 12 weeks, 6 months, and 1 year postoperatively. Preoperative standard anteroposterior (AP), lateral and oblique radiographs of the involved digit were assessed for joint narrowing, osteoporosis, subchondral erosions, joint ankylosis, and cyst formation. Joint reduction, subluxation, or dislocation were also documented. Evidence for axial subsidence, stem migration, resorption stress shielding, increasing radiolucent seam, periprosthetic erosions, and heterotopic bone formation was also evaluated.

Results

Of the 21 MP joints (19 patients) treated for OA with pyrolytic carbon (Ascension, Austin, Texas) arthroplasty, 20 were primary joint replacements and 1 was a revision following a fracture of a silicone implant. The average patient age was 57.2 years (range 31–75). Five patients (26.3%) were female and 14 (73.7%) were male. Twenty-six point three percent of patients admitted to smoking. The average duration of symptoms averaged 2.6 years (range 1–7 years). A history of direct trauma to the affected joint was recalled in 5 patients (26.3%). Five patients had undergone previous surgery on the affected joint before arthroplasty. At presentation, 100% of patients complained of pain with an average intensity of 75.2 on the visual analog scale (range 0–100). On average, patients felt their involved joint functioned only 23.1% of normal (Table 1). Goals of surgery, as reported by the patients, were pain control in 74%, improvement in function in 21%, and improvement in both pain and function in 5%.

Preoperative radiographic assessment showed that 43% of affected joints showed some evidence for subluxation; there were no cases of frank dislocation. Joint narrowing was noted in 85.7% of patients, subchondral erosion was noted in 57%, and heterotopic ossification was seen in 38% of patients. There were no cases of joint ankylosis.

A total of 10 index MP and 11 long-finger MP joints were treated. Concomitant procedures

Table 1
Range of motion and strength

ROM	MP flexion	MP ext (Lag)	Opp pinch (kg)	Grip (kg)	Bout	SN
Pre-op	65.5	21.1	1.4	20.3	0	0
6 weeks	63.2	11.2	NA	NA	0	0
12 weeks	66.1	14.2	3.3	23.4	0	0
6 months	69.1	12.7	2.2	30.4	0	0
1 year	73.2	15.2	3.2	28.1	0	0
% increase from pre-op	12.8	-28.0	125.9	38.2		

Abbreviations: Bout, boutonnière; ext, extension; Lag, extension deficit; NA, not available; Opp, oppositional; ROM, range of motion; SN, swan neck

included one intrinsic tendon release, four synovectomies, and two extensor tendon realignments. No intraoperative complications were noted.

The average duration of follow-up was 14 months (range 3–38.5). Range of motion (ROM) at the 1-year time point was expressed as a change from preoperative values. The preoperative average ROM was from minus 21° of extension to 65° of flexion at the MP joint. Postoperative, the average motion arc was seen to increase from minus 15° of extension to 73° of flexion. This represented a MP joint flexion increase of 12.8% ($P = 0.17$) and MP extension lag decrease of 28.0% ($P = 0.18$). Despite the improvement in motion, neither change reached significance. Final oppositional pinch increased 125.9% ($P = 0.02$) over preoperative values and grip strength improved nearly 40% ($P = 0.04$) (see Table 1). There were no cases of boutonnière or swan neck deformities developing during the postoperative follow-up.

All patients reported pain at initial presentation; this significantly declined throughout the postoperative course. Only 2 of the 19 patients noted any pain at 1 year. The analog pain scale averaged 73 preoperatively (scale 0 = no pain, 100 = worst pain possible) and 8.5 at final follow-up, an 88.4% decrease ($P = 0.0004$). The patients' grading for the functionality of the involved digit increased from 20.1% of normal anticipated function to a final value of 86.6%, an increase of 330.4% ($P = 0.0002$). Appearance of the digit was also felt to improve. Digital cosmesis approval rating rose from 62.7% to 93.6% at 1 year after surgery, an increase of 49.3 ($P = 0.01$) (Table 2).

Preoperatively, nine patients were working full-time, two part-time, two were on disability, four were retired, one unemployed, and one patient was a homemaker. At final follow-up, eight patients had returned to their preoperative work status (seven full-time, one part-time); one patient was able to regain full-time employment following arthroplasty. One patient in the study had remained retired and one became a student. Another patient retired from full-time work, but not because of disability or pain attributable to the surgery. A single patient remained on disability until lost to follow-up at the 1-year time point. Two patients are pending the 1-year follow-up, although one was retired at the time of surgery and the second had already returned to part-time employment by the 6-month mark. Data were not available on the four final patients: one homemaker, two retired preoperatively, and one employed full-time. In summary, 75% of patients returned to their previous employment status. In addition, one patient came out of retirement to regain full-time work status because of his improved function. Furthermore, one patient who

Table 2
Patient outcome measures

Group	Pain (% occurrence)	Analogue pain (% occurrence)	Function (% of normal)	Appearance (% of normal)	Satisfaction (% patients)
Pre-op	100	73.1	20.1	62.7	
6 weeks	31.6	8.9	68.3	81.2	100
12 weeks	15.8	7.1	78.3	86.1	100
6 months	10.5	11.8	75.3	82	94.7
1 year	10.5	8.5	86.6	93.6	94.7

did not return to full-time employment had re-tired, but not as a result of disability.

There were five (26.3%) complications; two were considered minor. One patient required extensor tendon suture removal at 6 weeks for irritation. A second patient developed MP joint swelling at 6 weeks because of joint capsule irritation, which resolved with extension splinting. There were three major complications: one case of extensor tendon rupture, one case of implant dislocation 4 months following surgery, and one case of chronic pain requiring implant removal. This last complication occurred in the index finger MP joint of a carpenter, who despite arthroplasty continued to complain of chronic pain inhibiting heavy labor. Re-exploration found no problem of wear present within the implant. Despite re-exploration, the patient eventually requested a ray amputation 1 year following initial surgery to allow him to continue his job as a carpenter. The patient continues to work full-time. Interest-ingly, of the three patients experiencing a major complication, all had had prior surgery on the involved joint and one patient had had surgery for revision of a fractured silicone implant. There did not appear to be any correlation between compli-cations and smoking status, medications, or past medical history.

Seven of the 19 total patients have been followed beyond 1 year, with an average post-operative assessment at 25 months (range 14–39). Within this group none reported pain. All patients had returned to their normal activities, including heavy labor employment and sport-related activ-ities such as golfing. All patients who had this long-term follow-up were very satisfied with their outcome.

Radiographic assessment

Radiographically, there was a single case of dislocation at 4 months following surgery. Peri-prosthetic erosion was noted in one patient at the 12-week follow-up and in 1 patient at the 1-year time point. The same patient who had the periprosthetic erosion at 1 year also represented the only case of resorption stress shielding seen at the 1-year mark. Despite radiographic findings, this patient has an excellent functional outcome and no pain.

An increase in the size of the radiolucent seam surrounding the implant is seen in all patients at 1-year follow-up, and in 62.5% of patients at 6-month follow-up. This appears to represent an incorporation of the implant stem into the sur-rounding bone, demonstrating a normal or antic-ipated radiolucent interface. Despite increase in seam size, none of the implants have demon-strated evidence of loosening or migration. There were no cases of axial subsidence, stem angular migration, heterotopic bone, or new cyst forma-tion within this series (Table 3) (Fig. 13).

Discussion

The functional demands on the MP joints in patients who have OA and TA can be much greater than those seen in RA patients. The use of constrained implants in these situations often results in high fracture rates or implant loosening. The use of unconstrained implants may represent a significant advantage for the young or active patient who has primary OA or TA involving the MP joint. In the authors' study we found pain relief to be excellent. Pinch and grip strength improved. In addition, approximately 60° of motion were maintained at the MP joint.

There are few long-term outcome studies focusing specifically on the role of surface re-placement arthroplasty in patients who have OA. The Ascension pyrolytic carbon implant achieved FDA approval in the United States in 2001; thus long-term studies are not yet in existence. Euro-pean trials have been ongoing, and experience with an earlier version of the implant has been previously reported [53,54]. Nuñez and Citron [54] performed a short-term outcome study focusing

Table 3
Radiographic outcomes

Post-op	Reduced %	Axial subsidence	Stem angular migration	Resorption stress shielding	Increased radiolucent seam	Periprosthetic erosions	Heterotopic bone	Cyst
6 week	100	0	0	0	0	0	0	0
12 week	100	0	0	0	9.5	4.8	0	0
6 months	94.1	0	0	0	62.5	0	0	0
1 year	100	0	0	9.1	100	9.1	0	0

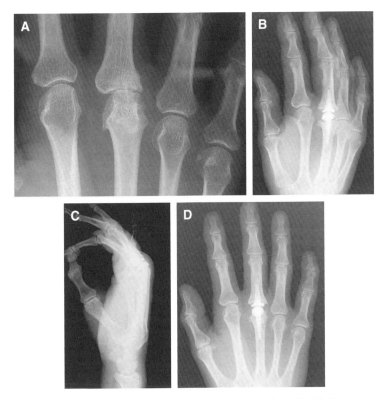

Fig. 13. (*A*) OA of the long-finger MP joint treated with pyrocarbon arthroplasty. (*B–D*) One-year postoperative radiographs show well-seated implant with congruent joint.

specifically the use of pyrolytic carbon implants in patients who had OA. Mean follow-up was 2.2 years. Results showed a significant improvement in pain with no cases of implant failure or loosening. Motion improved approximately 10° [54].

Cook and colleagues [53] reported their long-term outcome data on the use of pyrolytic carbon MP joint arthroplasty in 26 patients, the majority of who had RA. Average follow-up was 11.7 years. Results were encouraging, with a significant improvement in pain and a 13° increase in postoperative MP motion. Eighty-two percent of implants maintained their original postoperative reduced position. The majority of subluxations and dislocations occurred at greater then 10 years after implant placement [53].

Harris and Dias [55] reported their results with an unconstrained surface replacement arthroplasty placed primarily in an OA population. This implant consists of a metal metacarpal component and polyethylene distal component locked into uncemented polyethylene finned plugs. Five-year results in eight patients (seven of whom had OA) showed a 33° improvement in MP joint

ROM. One component was found to have settled, but there no cases of gross loosening [55].

Although pain relief was excellent in our study, improvement in finger ROM was modest. The 10° improvement in ROM is consistent with the previous findings of Cook and coworkers [53] and Nuñez and colleagues [54], but not as significant as those obtained by Harris and colleagues [55]. In all of these studies, patients have maintained approximately 50° to 60° of active pain-free motion. Cook and colleagues [53] also noted that the MP joints remain in a more extended position, allowing for an improvement in overall hand function. The authors feel that the return of pain-free motion was the major contributor to the improvement in pinch and grip strength seen in our patients. Similar improvements in strength were noted by Nuñez and coworkers [54].

Surface replacement inherently has less resistance to deforming forces of the extrinsic flexors and intrinsic muscles when compared with constrained implants; however, in the authors' series there was only a single case of dislocation and there were no cases of subluxation or radial or ulnar displacement. The one case of dislocation occurred following the use of a torque wrench at 4 months, and may represent an overly rapid advancement in this patient's hand activities. It was also encouraging to note that there were no cases of subsidence during the follow-up period. Significant subsidence has been linked to implant migration, joint space collapse, and periarticular heterotopic ossification and osteophyte formation [3,13,21]. The radiolucent seam seen in patients undergoing pyrocarbon arthroplasty is a consistent finding; this radiolucent shell should not be misinterpreted as loosening. This appears to represent an incorporation of the implant stem into the surrounding bone, demonstrating a normal or anticipated radiolucent interface. Despite increase in seam size, none of the implants have demonstrated evidence of loosening or migration.

Long-term studies have also found the rate of MP fracture to range from 6% to 47% [13]. In the authors' study, we saw no evidence of implant fracture, and in the Cook and coworkers study [53], only a single implant of 151 was noted to have fractures after 9 years, which attests to the biological compatibility and war resistance of this implant.

The most encouraging aspect of the surgery is the high rate of patient satisfaction. Despite the signal failure in this study, 94% of patients would have the surgery again, and have noted a significant improvement in finger function and cosmesis. Patients continue to comment that the motion produced by the pyrolytic carbon implant feels like a "normal joint."

Summary

Unconstrained pyrolytic surface replacement arthroplasty provides the benefits of a more natural center of rotation with preservation of native ligamentous joint stability. Initial short-term results show excellent motion, pain relief, and restoration of pinch and grip strength. These results are encouraging, and suggest that pyrolytic carbon arthroplasty may be a reasonable option for joint salvage in patients suffering from MP joint osteoarthritis.

References

[1] Brannon EW, Klein G. Experience with a finger-joint prosthesis. J Bone Joint Surg 1959;41:87–102.

[2] Flatt AE. Restoration of rheumatoid finger-joint function. Interim report on trial of prosthetic replacement. J Bone Joint Surg 1961;43:753–74.

[3] Doi K, Kuwata N, Kawai S. Alumina ceramic finger implants: a preliminary biomaterial and clinical evaluation. J Hand Surg [Am] 1984;9:740–9.

[4] Hagert CG, Branemark PI, Albrektsson T, et al. Metacarpophalangeal joint replacement with osseo-integrated endoprostheses. Scand J Plast Reconstr Surg 1986;20:207–18.

[5] Minami M, Yamazaki J, Kato S, et al. Alumina ceramic prosthesis arthroplasty of the metacarpophalangeal joint in the rheumatoid hand. A 2–4 year follow-up study. J Arthroplasty 1988;3:157–66.

[6] Varma SK, Milward TM. The Nicolle finger joint prosthesis: a reappraisal. J Hand Surg [Br] 1991;16B:187–90.

[7] Adams BD, Blair WF, Shurr DG. Schultz metacarpophalangeal arthroplasty: a long-term follow-up study. J Hand Surg [Am] 1990;15:641–5.

[8] Condamine JL, Benoit JY, Comtet JJ, et al. Proposed digital arthroplasty critical study of the preliminary results. Ann Chir Main 1988;7:282–97.

[9] Levack B, Stewart HD, Flierenga H, et al. Metacarpo-phalangeal joint replacement with a new prosthesis: description and preliminary results of treatment with the Helal flap joint. J Hand Surg [Br] 1987;12:377–81.

[10] Welsh RP, Hastings DE, White R. Resurfacing arthroplasty for the metacarpophalangeal joint. Acta Orthop Belg 1982;48:924–7.

[11] Wilson YG, Sykes PJ, Niranjan NS. Long-term follow-up of Swanson's silastic arthroplasty of the metacarpophalangeal joints in rheumatoid arthritis. J Hand Surg [Br] 1993;18:81–91.

[12] Beckenbaugh RD, Dobyns JH, Linscheid RL, et al. Review and analysis of silicone-rubber metacarpophalangeal implants. J Bone Joint Surg 1976;58:483–7.

[13] Blair WF, Shurr DG, Buckwalter JA. Metacarpophalangeal joint arthroplasty with a metallic hinged prosthesis. Clin Orthop 1984;184:156–63.

[14] Beckenbaugh RD. Pyrolytic carbon implants. In: Stanley J, Simmen BR, Allieu Y, et al, editors. Hand arthroplasties. London: Martin Dunitz; 2000. p. 323–7.

[15] Cook SD, Beckenbaugh RD, Weinstein AM, et al. Pyrolite carbon implants in the metacarpophalangeal joint of baboons. Orthopedics 1983;6:952–61.

[16] Beevers DJ, Seedhom BB. Metacarpophalangeal joint prosthesis. A review of the clinical results of past and current designs. J Hand Surg [Br] 1995;20:125–36.

[17] Hagert CG, Eiken O, Ohlsson NM, et al. Metacarpophalangeal joint implants: I. Roentgenographic study on the silastic finger joint implants. Swanson design. Scand J Plast Reconstr Surg 1975;9:147–57.

[18] Goldfarb CA, Stern PJ. Metacarpophalangeal joint arthroplasty in rheumatoid arthritis. J Bone Joint Surg 2003;85:1869–78.

[19] DeHeer DH, Owens SR, Swanson AB. The host response to silicone elastomer implants for small joint arthroplasty. J Hand Surg [Am] 1995;20: S101–9.

[20] Kay AG, Jeffs JV, Scott JT. Experience with silastic prosthesis in the rheumatoid hand. A 5-year follow-up. Ann Rheum Dis 1978;37:255–8.

[21] Kirschembaum D, Schneider LH, Adams DC, et al. Arthroplasty of the metacarpophalangeal joints with use of silicone-rubber implants in patients who have rheumatoid arthritis. Long-term results. J Bone Joint Surg 1993;75:3–12.

[22] Krishnan J, Chipchase L. Passive and axial rotation of the metacarpophalangeal joint. J Hand Surg [Br] 1997;22:270–3.

[23] Hakstian RW, Tubiana R. Ulnar deviation of the fingers. The role of joint structure and function. J Bone Joint Surg 1967;43:299–316.

[24] Long C. Intrinsic-extrinsic muscle control of the hand in power grip and precision handling. J Hand Surg [Am] 1970;22:286–98.

[25] Minami A, An KN, Cooney WP, et al. Ligament stability of the metacarpophalangeal joint: a biomechanical study. J Hand Surg [Am] 1985;10(2): 255–60.

[26] Gillespie TE, Flatt AE, Youm Y, et al. Biomechanical evaluation of metacarpophalangeal joint prosthesis designs. J Hand Surg [Am] 1979;4:508–21.

[27] Dubousset JF. Finger rotation during flexion. In: Tubiana R, editor. The hand. Philadelphia: WB Saunders; 1981. p. 202–6.

[28] Berme N, Paul JP, Purves WK. A biomechanical analysis of the metacarpophalangeal joint. J Biomech 1977;10:409–12.

[29] Youm Y, Gillespie TE, Flatt AE, et al. Kinematic investigation of the normal MCP joint. J Biomech 1978;11:109–18.

[30] Wise KS. The anatomy of the metacarpophalangeal joint with observations of the etiology of ulnar drift. J Bone Joint Surg 1975;57B:485.

[31] Tamai K, Ryu J, An KN, et al. Three dimensional geometric analysis of the metacarpophalangeal joint. J Hand Surg [Am] 1988;13:521–9.

[32] Pagowski S, Piekarski K. Biomechanics of the metacarpophalangeal joint. J Biomech 1977;10:205–9.

[33] Linscheid RL. Metacarpophalangeal arthroplasties: prosthetic design considerations. In: Stanley J, Simmen BR, Allieu Y, et al, editors. Hand arthroplasties. London: Martin Dunitz; 2000. p. 301–13.

[34] Linscheid RL. Implant arthroplasty of the hand; retrospective and prospective considerations. J Hand Surg [Am] 2000;25:796–816.

[35] Minami A, An KN, Cooney WP, et al. Ligamentous structures of the metacarpophalangeal joint: a quantitative anatomic study. J Orthop Res 1984;1(4): 361–8.

[36] Linscheid RL, Chao EY. Biomechanical assessment of finger function in prosthetic joint design. Orthop Clin North Am 1973;4:317–20.

[37] Linscheid RL, Dobyns JH. Total joint arthroplasty: the hand. Mayo Clin Proc 1979;54:227–40.

[38] Minamikawa Y, Imaeda T, Amadio PC, et al. Lateral stability of the proximal interphalangeal joint. J Hand Surg [Am] 1994;19:1050–4.

[39] McMaster M. The natural history of the rheumatoid metacarpophalangeal joint. J Bone Joint Surg 1972; 54B:687–97.

[40] Walker PS, Erkman MJ. Laboratory evaluation of a metal-plastic type of metacarpophalangeal joint prosthesis. Clin Orthop 1975;112:340–56.

[41] Schultz RJ, Storace A, Krishnamurthy S. Metacarpophalangeal joint motion and the role of the collateral ligament. Int Orthop 1987;11:149–55.

[42] Cooney WP. The future of hand and wrist joint replacement. In: Morrey B, editor. Joint replacement arthroplasty. New York: Churchill Livingston; 1991. p. 237–40.

[43] Smith EM, Juvinall RC, Bender LF, et al. Role of the finger flexors in rheumatoid deformities of the metacarpophalangeal joint. Arthritis Rheum 1964; 7:467–80.

[44] Flatt AE, Ellison MR. Restoration of rheumatoid finger joint function: 3. A follow-up note after fourteen years of experience with a metallic hinge prosthesis. J Bone Joint Surg 1972;54A:1317–22.

[45] Ellison MR, Flatt AE, Kelly KJ. Ulnar drift of the fingers in rheumatoid disease. J Bone Joint Surg 1971;53A:1061–82.

[46] Flatt AE, Fischer GW. Biomechanical factors in the replacement of rheumatoid finger joints. Ann Rheum Dis 1969;28:36–41.

[47] Smith RJ, Kaplan EB. Rheumatoid deformities at the metacarpophalangeal joints of the fingers. J Bone Joint Surg 1967;49A:31–47.

[48] Landsmeer JMF. The coordination of the finger joint motion. J Bone Joint Surg 1963;45A:1654–62.

[49] Chao EY, Opgrande JD, Axmear FE. Three-dimensional force analysis of finger joints in selected isometric hand functions. J Biomech 1976;9:387–96.

[50] An KN, Chao EY, Linscheid RL. Functional forces in normal and abnormal fingers. Orthopaed Trans 1978;2:168–70.

[51] An KN, Chao EY, Cooney WP, et al. Normative model of the human hand for biomechanical analysis. J Biomech 1979;12(10):775–8.

[52] An KN, Ueba Y, Chao EY, et al. Tendon excursion and moment arm of index finger muscle muscles. J Biomech 1983;16:419–25.

[53] Cook SD, Beckenbaugh RD, Redondo J, et al. Long-term follow-up of pyrocarbon metacarpophalangeal implants. J Bone Joint Surg 1999;81:635–47.

[54] Nuñez VA, Citron ND. Short-term results of Ascension pyrolytic carbon metacarpophalangeal joint replacement arthroplasty for osteoarthritis. Chir Main 2005;24:161–4.

[55] Harris D, Dias JJ. Five-year results of a new total replacement prosthesis for the finger metacarpophalangeal joints. J Hand Surg [Br] 2003;28:432–8.

ELSEVIER
SAUNDERS

Hand Clin 22 (2006) 195–200

HAND
CLINICS

Finger Metacarpophalangeal Joint Disease: The Role of Resection Arthroplasty and Arthrodesis

Matthew M. Tomaino, MD, MBA*, Michael Leit, MD

University of Rochester Medical Center, 601 Elmwood Ave, Box 665, Rochester, NY 14642, USA

When it comes to arthrosis of the finger metacarpophalangeal (MP) joint, implant arthroplasty is, for the most part, the treatment of choice when pain or instability impair function. Indeed, functional grasp, particularly of the ulnar three digits, relies on flexion at the MP joint. In the setting of post-traumatic or postinfectious disease, however, alternative techniques of restoring pain-free function become relevant. The authors' purpose in this article is to discuss the limited roles of resection arthroplasty and arthrodesis when implant arthroplasty may be contraindicated.

Kinematic and biomechanical considerations

Active ranges of motion of the joints of the hand are well-documented, but there are few data reporting the functional ranges of motion required to perform activities of daily living. Using electrogoniometric and standard methods Hume and colleagues [1] measured both active and functional ranges of motion of the metacarpophalangeal (MP) and interphalangeal (IP) joints during 11 activities of daily living. In the fingers, only a small percentage of the active range of motion of the joints was required for functional tasks. Functional flexion postures averaged 61° at the MP joint, 60° at the proximal interphalangeal (PIP) joint, and 39° at the distal interphalangeal (DIP) joint [1].

Beyond classifying finger movement based on the final position of the hand, Nakamura and

coworkers [2] have provided a description of the movement process at each of the three finger joints, using measurements and analysis from a two-dimensional motion analyzer. They examined the grasping of discs of different diameter in 15 healthy volunteers, and found that joint movement was initiated from distal to proximal, but the final motion for grasping was carried to completion from the proximal to distal joints of the finger in most subjects. In addition, it was recognized that the proportion of the angular change in each of the three joints was different, as were the time duration of the joint motion and the pattern of the angular change [2].

Indeed, it appears that deliberate activities of the finger and sophisticated joint movements provide delicate adjustments to fit the fingers to the size of an object, and that the PIP joint is perhaps most instrumental in initiating such movement [3].

Lee and Rim [4] measured finger joint angles and forces during maximal cylindrical grasping, and found that finger flexion angles at the MP and PIP joints gradually increase as cylinder diameter decreases, but that at the DIP joint the angle remains constant throughout all cylinder sizes. They also found that total finger force increases as cylinder size decreases [4].

Coordinated action of the extrinsic flexors during finger flexion contributes importantly to the linked motions of the IP joints, but the actions of the intrinsic muscles are necessary for stabilizing the MP joint in flexion postures during IP motion and in producing motions voluntarily limited to the MP joint [5]. This suggests that stabilization of the MP joint is required for the rest of the finger to be effective. Thus, in the absence of functional intrinsics and capsuloligamentous

* Corresponding author.

E-mail address: matthew_tomaino@urmc.rochester.edu (M.M. Tomaino).

0749-0712/06/$ - see front matter © 2006 Elsevier Inc. All rights reserved.
doi:10.1016/j.hcl.2006.02.011

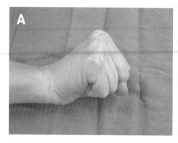
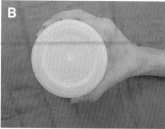
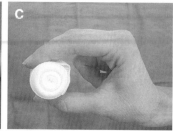

Fig. 1. (*A*) Clenched fist reveals more MP joint flexion at the ring and small finger than index and long. (*B*) Grasping a cylindrical object shows similar MP flexion at each MP joint. (*C*) Prehension between thumb, index, and long requires about 30° of MP flexion.

restraints, impairment of coordinated IP joint function is likely.

Clinical considerations

Scrutiny of one's own hand in varying stages of grasp reveals that the position of the MP joint at the extreme of making a fist becomes more flexed moving from index to small. Index and long MP joints assume less of a flexion posture than ring and small, and for most types of prehension that require either key or chuck pinch, the radial MP joints flex no more than 30° or so (Fig. 1).

In terms of grasping a cylindrical object, only those with extremely small circumferences require any of the finger MP joints to flex more than this amount (see Fig. 1). And, as was highlighted above, despite the modest flexion required at the

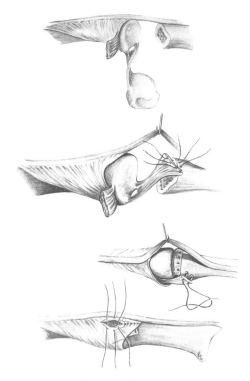

Fig. 2. Tupper arthroplasty, in which the distally based volar plate is used for resurfacing. (*From* Flatt AE. Care of the arthritic hand. 4th edition. Philadelphia: Mosby; 1983; with permission.)

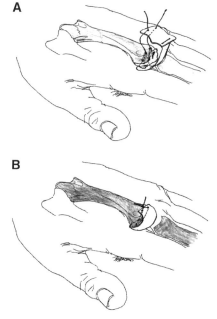

Fig. 3. (*A*) Horizontal mattress suture is preplaced through drill holes in the metacarpal. (*B*) The suture is tied down and the graft conforms to the shape of the metacarpal. (*From* Netscher D, Eladoumikdachi F, Gao YH. Resurfacing arthroplasty for metacarpophalangeal joint osteoarthritis: a good option using either perichondrium or extensor retinaculum. Plast Reconstr Surg 2000;106:1430–3; with permission.)

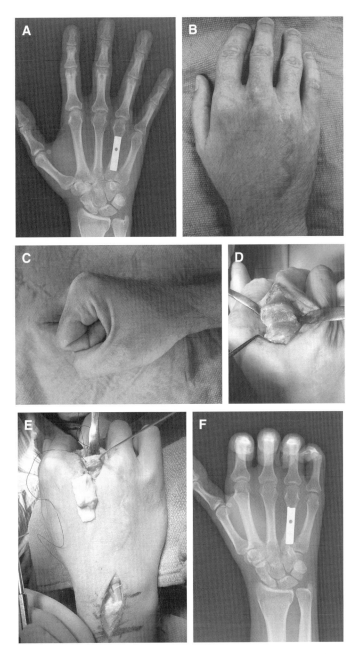

Fig. 4. Resection arthroplasty case example: (*A*) Preoperative posteroanterior (PA) radiograph shows MP joint arthrosis. (*B*) Preoperative photograph of the dorsum of the hand. (*C*) Preoperative flexion. (*D*) Intraoperative photograph of the resected MP joint. (*E*) Intraoperative photograph of the harvested extensor retinaculum. (*F*) Postoperative PA radiograph 6 months following surgery. (*G*) Flexion 6 months after resection arthroplasty. (*H*) Extension 6 months after resection arthroplasty.

MP joint for most grasping activities, stability is essential to empower, if you will, the rest of the finger, particularly the PIP joint.

Arthrosis of the finger MP joints is not uncommon, and is usually secondary to inflammatory arthritis. In general, such problems are commonly amenable to implant arthroplasty; however, in the setting of postinfectious arthrosis or following trauma, in which soft-tissue restraints or bone are absent, alternative reconstructive techniques must

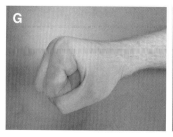 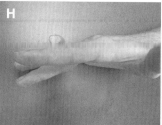

Fig. 4 (*continued*)

be used. Resection arthroplasty and arthrodesis may provide valuable salvage.

Resection arthroplasty

This salvage should be reserved for the failed implant arthroplasty, when there is a history of sepsis, in cases where bone stock is inadequate to provide implant fixation, or when soft tissue is deficient to provide implant stability. The principles of resection arthroplasty include sufficient bone resection to correct deformity and permit motion, and resurfacing or tissue interposition to prevent painful impingement or autofusion.

Though use of rib perichondrium has been described [6], it probably provides little advantage over other techniques with potentially less morbidity. Seradge and colleagues [6] reported on 16 MP joint perichondrial resurfacing arthroplasties, and showed an average total range of motion of only 22°. Further, in patients older than 30, unsatisfactory results were common.

A variety of techniques of resection arthroplasty have been described. Resurfacing has used fascia lata [7]; extensor tendon, as described by Vainio [8]; volar plate, as described by Tupper [9]; and extensor retinaculum [10]. From a practical standpoint, fascia lata harvest is not recommended, given the feasibility of alternative techniques, although use of allograft might be reasonable except for the added expense. The Tupper arthroplasty [9] is less likely to result in an MP joint extensor lag than when the extensor tendon [8] is used for interposition, but length of the volar plate may limit the amount of flexion that is possible after suturing it to the dorsal metacarpal surface (Fig. 2).

The authors prefer use of a relatively new technique described by Netscher and coworkers [10], which uses extensor retinaculum (Fig. 3). The

contour of the metacarpal head is maintained, providing, at least in theory, a more congruous arc of motion.

Case example

A 25-year-old man had been involved in a fight 8 months earlier, when he sustained a tooth cut to the long MP joint. He subsequently required surgical debridement and antibiotic treatment for septic arthritis. He presented with limited motion, pain, and radiographic evidence of MP joint arthrosis (Fig. 4). His primary complaints included pain and insufficient flexion. The authors performed resection arthroplasty using the technique described by Netscher and colleagues [10], using extensor retinaculum. Six months following surgery, the patient was pleased with functional outcome and pain relief.

Metacarpophalangeal joint arthrodesis

Arthrodesis of the finger MP joint is most specifically indicated in preference to resection arthroplasty for isolated joint arthrosis in the border digits (index or small) or in a manual laborer. A position of 20° to 30° has been recommended [11]. In general, however, a procedure that retains some motion is preferable; however, when stability and pain relief at the MP joint are provided by fusion, functional patterns of prehension can be restored (see Fig. 1). In the absence of ligamentous support, appropriate bone stock, and intrinsic function, arthrodesis is clearly a better option than a motion-preserving procedure (Fig. 5).

Though fusion can be performed with Kirshner wires or plates and screws, the authors have been satisfied of late with the use of staples (OSStaple, BioMedical Enterprises, San Antonio,

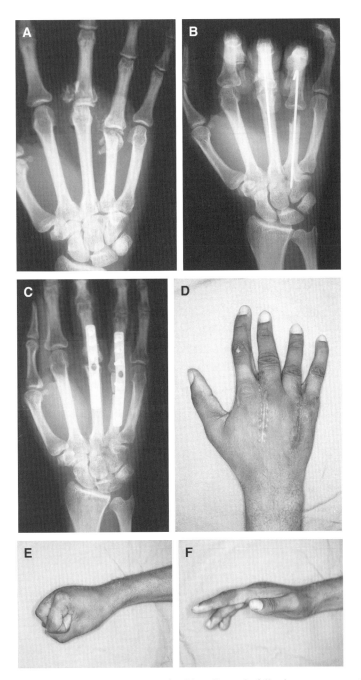

Fig. 5. MP joint Arthrodesis case example: (*A*) Preoperative PA radiographs following open trauma to the long and ring finger MP joints, and (*B*) after irrigation, debridement, and provisional stabilization. (*C*) PA radiograph following long and ring MP joint arthrodesis. (*D*) Postoperative finger flexion, (*E*) finger flexion, and (*F*) finger extension.

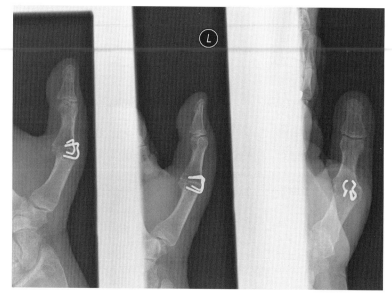

Fig. 6. Postoperative radiographs after thumb MP joint arthrodesis with the use of staples.

Texas), not only at the MP joint, but at the carpometacarpal joint as well (Fig. 6).

Summary

When finger MP joint arthrosis exists, it is indeed infrequent that implant arthroplasty is not the most optimal treatment alternative. When post-traumatic bone loss or postinfectious dysfunction require surgical intervention, however, the hand surgeon may need to consider the options of resection arthroplasty and arthrodesis. So long as the MP joint is pain-free and relatively stable, most patterns of functional prehension can be maintained.

References

[1] Hume MC, Gellman H, Mckellop H, et al. Functional range of motion of the joints of the hand. J Hand Surg [Am] 1990;15:240–3.

[2] Nakamura M, Miyawaki C, Matsushita N, et al. Analysis of voluntary finger movements during hand tasks by a motion analyzer. J Electromyogr Kinesiol 1998;8:295–303.

[3] Holguin PH, Rico AA, Gomez LP, et al. The coordinate movement of the interphalangeal joints. A cinematic study. Clin Orthop Relat Res 1999;362: 117–24.

[4] Lee JW, Rim K. Measurement of finger joint angles and maximum finger forces during cylinder grip activity. J Biomed Eng 1991;13:152–62.

[5] Darling WG, Cole KJ, Miller GF. Coordination of index finger movements. J Biomech 1994;27:479–91.

[6] Seradge H, Kutz JA, Kleinert HE, et al. Perichondrial resurfacing arthroplasty in the hand. J Hand Surg [Am] 1984;9:880–6.

[7] Fowler SB. Arthroplasty of the metacarpophalangeal joint in rheumatoid arthritis. J Bone Joint Surg 1962;44:1037.

[8] Vainio K. Vainio arthroplasty of the metacarpophalangeal joints in rheumatoid arthritis. J Hand Surg [Am] 1989;14:367–8.

[9] Tupper JW. The metacarpophalangeal volar plate arthroplasty. J Hand Surg [Am] 1989;14:371–5.

[10] Netscher D, Eladoumikdachi F, Gao YH. Resurfacing arthroplasty for metacarpophalangeal joint osteoarthritis: a good option using either perichondrium or extensor retinaculum. Plast Reconstr Surg 2000; 106:1430–3.

[11] Moberg E. Arthrodesis of finger joints. Surg Clin North Am 1960;40:465–70.

ELSEVIER
SAUNDERS

Hand Clin 22 (2006) 201–206

HAND
CLINICS

Prosthetic Replacement of the Proximal Interphalangeal Joint

Peter M. Murray, MD[a,b,*]

[a]Department of Orthopaedic Surgery, Mayo Clinic College of Medicine,
200 1st Street SW, Rochester, MN 55905, USA
[b]Department of Orthopaedic Surgery, Division of Education, Mayo Clinic, 4500 San Pablo Road,
Jacksonville, FL 32224, USA

In 1940, Burman reported the use of a Vitallium cap for proximal interphalangeal joint (PIPJ) arthroplasty [1]. This and other early digital implants used concepts similar to those used in the highly successful implant arthroplasty of the lower extremity. In 1959, Brannon and Klein [2] from Lackland Air Force Base, Texas published the first series of a digital total joint replacement. They reported encouraging results with the use of a hinged prosthesis initially used for traumatic PIPJ injuries. Two years later, Flatt [3] reported on the use of a more rotationally stable form of the Brannon prosthesis. This prosthesis was indicated in patients who had arthritis [3,4].

In 1979, Linscheid and Dobyns developed a prototype of a PIPJ prosthesis, which they termed "surface replacement arthroplasty (SRA)." This prosthesis intended to preserve the collateral ligaments and unload the component stems [5]. Various modifications of this prosthesis have occurred with the most recent modification referred to as the PIP-SRA (Avanta, SBI, New York, New York). Subsequently, a variety of designs were developed including the Keesler, the Hagert, and the Sibly-Unsworth [4,6].

Biomechanics and prosthetic design

Restoring motion and alleviating pain are the primary goals of PIPJ replacement arthroplasty. Because of early design failures, total joint arthroplasty for the PIPJ has been slow to develop. These first-generation hinged designs failed because of nonanatomic centers of rotation, a high hinge mechanism coefficient of friction, metallic implant debris, and ultimately breakage [5,6]. A second generation of hinged prostheses was developed with a "ball and socket" design, attempting to add adduction and abduction motion to flexion and extension [6]. These designs were fraught with complications, including proximal phalangeal component failure, hypertrophic bone formation, poor motion, and instability [5,7].

The principal shortcoming of previous metallic or metalloplastic hinged designs has been the amount of bone resection needed for implantation. The primary stabilizing factors of the PIPJ is the bicondylar geometry of the articulation and the radial and ulnar collateral ligaments [8,9]. The extensor mechanism is also considered a stabilizer [8,9]. The bone resection required for insertion of the first and second generation devices violated the origin and insertion of the PIPJ collateral ligaments. The monoaxial hinged design of the first generation PIPJ arthroplasty created high loads borne by the component stems. Loosening, cortical penetration, and subsidence were among the complications encountered [2–4,6,8,10]. Subsequent constrained linked designs were unable to improve on these shortcomings.

The newest generation of PIPJ arthroplasty can be termed "surface replacement arthroplasty." The rationale behind this design is that a minimally constrained, unlinked prosthesis with an anatomic center of rotation can better balance forces acting across the joint. Preserving bone stock and

---

* Department of Orthopaedic Surgery, Mayo Clinic, 4500 San Pablo Road, Jacksonville, FL 32224.
E-mail address: murray.peter@mayo.edu

collateral ligament origins and insertions enhances stability of the arthroplasty. This stability is particularly important when index and long finger PIPJ arthroplasty is considered. Sustained pinch forces of over 70N are often encountered between the thumb and index fingers and the thumb and ring fingers. Resultant forces on the PIPJ can be as high as six times this sustained, externally applied force [6]. A successful arthroplasty, therefore, must withstand these transmitted forces. In theory, greater durability from the surface replacement arthroplasty can be expected compared with previous hinged designs. The anatomic configuration of the prosthesis and the retention of the collateral ligaments and PIPJ capsule should reduce axial torque at the bone/prosthesis interface [8]. Ash and Unsworth [11] have demonstrated that an anatomically designed PIPJ surface replacement arthroplasty could withstand pinch forces in excess of 65N. They have also shown that an ultra-high molecular weight polyethylene material for both weight- bearing surfaces could produce wear rates similar to metal on polymer [11].

One such PIPJ surface replacement implant (SBI), has a stemmed, bicondylar proximal phalangeal component milled from a CoCr alloy. The middle phalangeal component of this PIPJ implant is machined from ultra-high-molecular–weight polyethylene. The polyethylene articular surface is supported by a thin titanium backing and a broad stem. The articular surfaces of the proximal and middle phalangeal components are matched and are congruent. The component stems are designed to fit the internal contours of the medullary canal. The low profile design of the PIPJ surface replacement arthroplasty requires less bone removal, thereby preserving the integrity of the lateral collateral ligaments (Figs. 1, 2A–C).

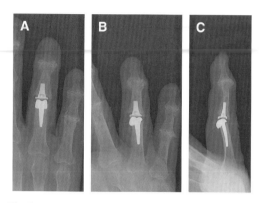

Fig. 2. (A, B, C) 87-year-old male with PIPJ osteoarthritis treated with SBI/Avanta surface replacement arthroplasty of the right ring finger.

Based on anthropomorphic data, four component sizes have been made. Currently, the PIPJ surface replacement arthroplasty is approved for advanced osteoarthritis, post-traumatic arthritis, and for revision arthroplasty of the PIPJ. Use of this prosthesis is less desirable in settings of pronounced bone loss or where the collateral ligaments are incompetent.

The Ascension PIP joint prosthetic replacement (Ascension Orthopedics, Austin, Texas) is a pyrolytic carbon implant with an anatomic design (Fig. 3). The device is indicated for implantation in patients with osteoarthritis or post-traumatic arthritis of the PIP joint. The pyrolytic carbon is a coating material formed by heating propane to 1300° Celsius. The hydrocarbon gas is then applied to a graphite substrate to create the pyrocarbon implant [12]. Two attractive features of pyrocarbon are an elastic modulus similar to cortical bone, creating a favorable situation for load transfer; and a low incidence of wear debris or soft-tissue reaction [13].

Other newer designs have focused more on improved intermedullary fixation rather than anatomic configuration of the articular surfaces [5,14,15]. These designs include the Saffar (Dimso

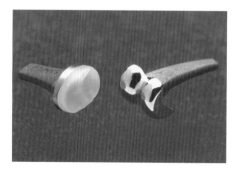

Fig. 1. Small Bone Innovations PIPJ surface replacement arthroplasty. (Courtesy of Avanta Orthopedics/ Small Bone Innovations, New York, NY.)

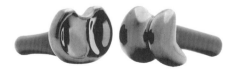

Fig. 3. Ascension PIPJ pyrolytic carbon implant. (Courtesy of Ascension Orthopedics, Austin, TX.)

S.A., Mernande, France), the Digitos (Osteo A.G., Selzach, Switzerland), the DJOA3 (Landos, Chaumont, France) and the Wecko Finger- grundgelenk prosthesis (Implant Service, Ham- burg, Germany). The Saffar and the DJOA3 prosthesis have a prominent stabilizing midline crest between the proximal and distal components and are considered "semiconstrained" by the manufacturers. The DJOA3 (Fig. 4) is composed of a stainless steel proximal component and a polyethylene distal component. Insertion of the prosthesis does not require preservation of the collateral ligaments. The Saffar prosthesis has a similar design that includes a noncemented, semiconstrained, titanium-polyethylene prosthesis [5]. The modular Digitos prosthesis (Fig. 5) is a fully constrained prosthesis designed specifically for unstable joints missing the collateral liga- ments. In essence, it is a second-generation device. Similarly, the Wecko Fingergrundgelenk prosthe- sis is a constrained design that fits into the inter- medullary bone sleeve (Fig. 6).

Technique of proximal interphalangeal joint arthroplasty

Different surgical approaches have been used for the various PIPJ prosthetic devices, including dorsal, lateral, and palmar approaches [8]. Because important structures must be negotiated with all these approaches, postoperative difficulties may occur. With the dorsal approach, the central slip is vulnerable; and with the lateral approach, the collateral ligaments are at risk. The volar plate and the flexor tendon sheath are at risk with the volar or anterior approach. Linscheid and

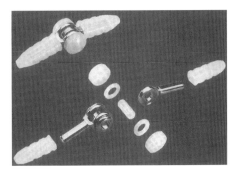

Fig. 5. The DIGITOS PIPJ prosthesis. (*From* Linscheid RL. Implant arthroplasty of the hand: retrospective and prospective considerations. J Hand Surg [Am] 2000;25:796–816; with permission from the American Society for Surgery of the Hand.)

colleagues [8] reported late swan-neck deformities in patients undergoing PIPJ surface replacement arthroplasty when the palmar approach was used. Lin and colleagues [16], however, reported no instances of swan-neck deformity or flexor ten- don bowstring with the palmar approach used in 69 silicone arthroplasties [16]. Currently the author's preferred approach for the PIPJ surface replacement is the modified dorsal approach described by Chamay [17]. This approach offers extensile exposure of the PIPJ through a distally based triangular flap of the extensor mechanism (Fig. 7). Remnants of the dorsal PIPJ capsule are also identified and incised. The radial and ulnar collateral ligaments are protected using small

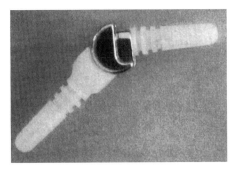

Fig. 4. The DJOA3 PIPJ prosthesis. (*From* Linscheid RL. Implant arthroplasty of the hand: retrospective and prospective considerations. J Hand Surg [Am] 2000;25:796–816; with permission from the American Society for Surgery of the Hand.)

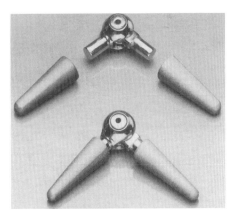

Fig. 6. The Wecko Fingergrundgelenk PIPJ prosthesis. (*From* Linscheid RL. Implant arthroplasty of the hand: retrospective and prospective considerations. J Hand Surg [Am] 2000;25:796–816; with permission from the American Society for Surgery of the Hand.)

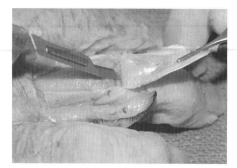

Fig. 7. Dorsal Chamay approach for PIPJ surface re-placement arthroplasty.

Homan retractors, also bringing the articular surface of the middle phalanx into view.

For PIPJ arthroplasty performed through the dorsal approach, an osteotomy of the base of the middle phalanx is made perpendicular to its long axis. For surface replacement arthroplasty, the collateral ligament insertions are protected, although a small portion of the insertion may be undermined [18]. Minamikawa and coworkers [9] have shown in a cadaver model that the PIPJ remains stable following removal of 50% of the collateral ligament substance. Following preparation of the middle phalanx base, the proximal phalangeal head is prepared by an osteotomy accomplished just proximal to the articular surface (Fig. 8). This is done perpendicular to the long axis of the proximal phalanx, and while protecting the proximal origin of the radial and ulnar collateral ligaments. A small burr is then used to shape the resected proximal phalangeal head to accept the desired prosthetic device. For insertion of the PIPJ surface replacement arthroplasty, this requires the creation of a "chamfer" back cut, so

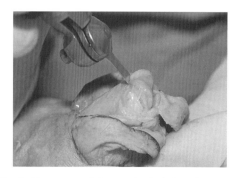

Fig. 8. Osteotomy of the proximal phalanx just proximal to the articular surface.

the proximal phalanx can accept the proximal component. The proximal and middle phalanges are then appropriately broached and trial components inserted. Once sizing for "best fit" is completed, the permanent components are implanted employing a "press-fit" technique. The extensor mechanism is repaired with 3-0 Surgilon suture.

If the dorsal approach is used, a controlled rehabilitation protocol is needed to prevent central slip failure. The rehabilitation program is initiated by postoperative day 5 under most circumstances. A dynamic extension splint permitting active flexion and dynamic extension is applied for 6 weeks during the day, and a static, forearm-based digital extension splint is used at night. During the first 2 weeks, the patient is limited to a 30° flexion block, followed by a 60° block at 4 weeks. By 6 weeks, all splints are discontinued and unrestricted flexion and extension is permitted.

Silastic athroplasty

In the early 1970s the design for the metacarpophalangeal (MCP) silastic implant was modified to accommodate the smaller canal size of the distal proximal phalanx and the middle phalanx. These devices were made from a relatively strong, non-reactive rubber polymer. The hinged silastic spacer remains the most common implant for PIPJ reconstruction, particularly in the rheumatoid patient, in whom 90% 10-year survivorship has been reported [19,20]; however, silastic implant arthroplasty is generally not recommended for the index or long fingers, particularly in active individuals [18,21]. The bony resection required for the proximal phalangeal head sacrifices the PIPJ radial and ulnar collateral ligaments, thereby causing the silastic to become vulnerable to the high loads seen during the pinching maneuver.

For silastic PIPJ arthroplasty, a volar approach is often used with a standard Brunner incision. The A-3 pulley is excised and the flexor tendons are retracted to expose the volar plate, which is detached proximally off the proximal phalanx. The collateral ligaments are released and the PIPJ hyperextended, much like a shotgun, to expose the articular surfaces of the proximal and middle phalanges. The proximal phalangeal head is excised with an oscillating saw. The base of the middle phalanx is not resected to avoid postoperative collapse deformity of the digit. The intramedullary canals are prepared with broaches. Rotational malalignment is specifically avoided.

Trial components are sized and a trial reduction performed. Once a satisfactory implant has been chosen, the permanent prosthesis is placed and the PIPJ reduced. Grommets are not used. The collateral ligaments are reattached to the proximal phalanx, if possible. This is not always feasible. The volar plate can be split longitudinally and used to reconstruct the collateral ligaments. Ideally, the volar plate should be repaired and the original collateral ligaments reattached. After the first week postoperative, the patient is placed in an extension outrigger splint, and active flexion and passive extension are initiated with a flexion block. The degree of flexion permitted is gradually increased, such that the extension outrigger splint is discontinued at 4 weeks postoperative. The operative digit is then buddy-taped to the adjacent digit for up to 3 months.

Results

The Swanson silicone PIPJ implant has been extensively evaluated. Ashworth and colleagues [19] reported on PIPJ silicone implants at an average follow-up of 5.8 years. Pain was not present in 67%, and at 9 years, prosthesis survivorship was 81%. The average postoperative arc of motion was 29°, compared with an average preoperative arc of motion of 38°. There were few complications in this series. Similarly, Lin and coworkers [16] reported on 69 silicone PIPJ spacers (48 with primary or post-traumatic osteoarthritis) at a mean follow-up of 3.4 years. The postoperative range of motion was 46°, compared with 44° preoperative. The average preoperative extension deficit was 17°, compared with 8° postoperative. Sixty-seven of the 69 patients were relieved of pain. There were 12 joints with complications in this series, including five implant fractures. Most surgeons do not advocate the use of silicone spacers in the index or long PIP joints of active individuals. This is because of the high potential pinch force loads seen at the index and long finger PIP joints (Fig. 9).

Initial results using the surface replacement PIPJ (SBI) were published by Linscheid and colleagues in 1997 [8]. In this study, 66 PIPJ surface replacement arthroplasties were performed, with the majority of digits having osteoarthritis. After a mean follow-up of 4.5 years, 32 joints had good results, 19 fair, and 25 poor. This series included results from earlier versions of the surface replacement design. Better results were obtained from arthroplasties performed through

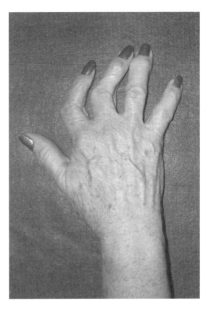

Fig. 9. Silicone spacer failures at the PIPJ of the index and long in a 67-year-old female.

a dorsal approach than those performed through a lateral or palmar approach. Complications occurred in 19 of the 66 PIPJ arthroplasties, and included instability, ulnar deviation, swan-neck deformity, flexion contracture, tenodesis, and joint subluxation. Component loosening was not observed. Range of motion at follow-up averaged from −14° extension to 61° flexion. There was a 12° in flexion/extension arc compared with the preoperative status [8].

Published results are not available for the Saffar and the Digitos prosthetic devices. Condamine and colleagues [14] have reported the results of the DJOA3, which they consider a "third-generation" PIPJ prosthetic device (see Fig. 4). The study reported satisfactory function in 110 implanted prostheses, with only a 3% loosening rate; however, 80% of the patients in this series had been followed for less than 1 year.

References

[1] Burman MS. Vitallium cap arthroplasty of metacarpophalangeal and interpalangeal joints of fingers. Bull Hospital Joints Dis 1940;1:79–89.

[2] Brannon EW, Klein G. Experiences with a finger-joint prosthesis. J Bone Joint Surg Am 1959;41-A: 87–102.

[3] Flatt A. Restoration of rheumatoid finger-joint function: interim report on trial of prosthetic replacement. J Bone Joint Surg Am 1961;43A:753–74.

[4] Beevers DJ, Seedhom BB. Metacarpophalangeal joint prostheses. A review of the clinical results of past and current designs. J Hand Surg [Br] 1995; 20:125–36.

[5] Linscheid RL. Implant arthroplasty of the hand: retrospective and prospective considerations. J Hand Surg [Am] 2000;25:796–816.

[6] Beevers DJ, Seedhom BB. Metacarpophalangeal joint prostheses: a review of past and current designs. Proc Inst Mech Eng [H] 1993;207:195–206.

[7] Adams BD, Blair WF, Shurr DG. Schultz metacarpophalangeal arthroplasty: a long-term follow-up study. J Hand Surg [Am] 1990;15:641–5.

[8] Linscheid RL, Murray PM, Vidal MA, et al. Development of a surface replacement arthroplasty for proximal interphalangeal joints. J Hand Surg [Am] 1997;22:286–98.

[9] Minamikawa Y, Horii E, Amadio PC, et al. Stability and constraint of the proximal interphalangeal joint. J Hand Surg [Am] 1993;18:198–204.

[10] Flatt AE, Ellison MR. Restoration of rheumatoid finger joint function. 3. A follow-up note after fourteen years of experience with a metallic-hinge prosthesis. J Bone Joint Surg Am 1972;54:1317–22.

[11] Ash HE, Unsworth A. Design of a surface replacement prosthesis for the proximal interphalangeal joint. Proc Inst Mech Eng [H] 2000;214:151–63.

[12] Cook SD, Beckenbaugh RD, Redondo J, et al. Long-term follow-up of pyrolytic carbon metacarpophalangeal implants. J Bone Joint Surg Am 1999;81:635–48.

[13] Cook SD, Beckenbaugh RD, Weinstein A, et al. Pyrolite carbon implants in the metacarpophalangeal joint of baboons. Orthopedics 1983;6:952–61.

[14] Condamine J, Marcucci L, Bisson P, et al. DJOA arthroplasty: ten years experience and introducing the DJOA 3. In: Schuind F, Cooney WP, An K-N, et al, editors. Advances in biomechanics of the hand and wrist. New York: Plenum Press; 1996. p. 76–83.

[15] Saffar P. La fixation prothetique: generalities. Table ronde sur les prosthesies interphalangiennes proximales: Congres de la Societe Francaise de Chirurgie de la Main [The fixation of prosthetic implants. Round table discussion of prosthetic implants of the proximal phalanx. Proceedings of the Congress of the French Society for Surgery of the Hand, Paris France]; 1997:107–9.

[16] Lin HH, Wyrick JD, Stern PJ. Proximal interphalangeal joint silicone replacement arthroplasty: clinical results using an anterior approach. J Hand Surg [Am] 1995;20:123–32.

[17] Chamay A. A distally based dorsal and triangular tendinoous flap for direct access to the proximal interphalangeal joint. Ann Chir Main 1988;179–83.

[18] Berger RA. Arthroplasty in the hand and wrist. In: Green DP, editor. Operative hand surgery. New York: Churchill Livingstone; 1999. p. 147–91.

[19] Ashworth CR, Hansraj KK, Todd AO, et al. Swanson proximal interphalangeal joint arthroplasty in patients with rheumatoid arthritis. Clin Orthop Relat Res 1997;342:34–7.

[20] Hansraj KK, Ashworth CR, Ebramzadeh E, et al. Swanson metacarpophalangeal joint arthroplasty in patients with rheumatoid arthritis. Clin Orthop Relat Res 1997;342:11–5.

[21] Linscheid RL, Dobyns JH. Total joint arthroplasty. The hand. Mayo Clin Proc 1979;54:516–26.

ELSEVIER
SAUNDERS

Hand Clin 22 (2006) 207–210

Distal Interphalangeal Joint Arthrodesis with Screw Fixation: Why and How

Matthew M. Tomaino, MD, MBA

University of Rochester Medical Center, 601 Elmwood Avenue, Box 665, Rochester, NY 14642, USA

Arthrodesis of the distal interphalangeal (DIP) joint is a common procedure to treat the painful, unstable distal joint in the osteoarthritic and rheumatoid patient. Less common indications include chronic mallet deformity, missed flexor digitorum profundus avulsions, and distal middle phalangeal fracture nonunion. In most cases, successful fusion improves digital function. Morbidity—to the extent that any elective procedure needs to balance the pros and cons—stems from wound healing problems, infection, and painful nonunion. Though Burton and colleagues [1] advocated the use of Kirschner wires (K-wires) alone, reporting a nonunion rate for the small joints of the hand of .6%, wires at the DIP joint, in particular, are frequently a nuisance—they get caught on clothing, get infected, and may back out or fall out altogether. Indeed, Stern and Fulton [2] reported a 20% complication rate, including hardware protrusion or migration, loosening, failure to achieve union, pin track infections, and stiffness. Though nonunion rate did not differ between technical alternatives, buried hardware avoided some of the others.

Based on the expectation that compression across the DIP joint might accelerate fusion, both the Herbert (Zimmer, Warsaw, Indiana) [3–5] and the Mini-Acutrak (Acumed, Beaverton, Oregon) screws have proven successful [6]. The author prefers the Herbert screw over the newer cannulated screws because it is less expensive, is just as easy to insert, and allows manual compression after placement, in the event that the bony surfaces are not entirely coapted after screw placement.

E-mail address: matthew_tomaino@urmc.rochester.edu

Surgical technique

Under regional anesthesia, a dorsal bayonet-shaped incision is made, and skin flaps are elevated off the extensor tendon. The tendon is divided transversely, the joint is flexed, and the collateral ligaments are released. Beginning with the head of the middle phalanx, a small rongeur is used to trim dorsal osteophytes. Next the articular surface is removed, leaving the remaining decorticated surface flat relative to the orientation of the shaft. Now, with improved exposure of the base of the distal phalanx, the rongeur is used to decorticate the base of P-3, preserving as much bone stock as possible.

A .045 K-wire is drilled antegrade through the base of P-3 out the finger tip, just deep to the nail bed. This allows the narrower Herbert drill bit, which corresponds to the leading edge of the Herbert screw, to be passed by hand, antegrade, through the same path. When it presses up the skin distally as it exits, a small incision is made. This same narrow drill bit is passed retrograde through the head of P-2 to about midway down the shaft. Next, the larger diameter drill bit, which corresponds to the trailing head of the screw, is passed retrograde through the fingertip incision, into the tip of P-3, until its hub prevents further passage. Starting this bit requires "catching" the exit hole at the tip of P-3, which had been made by the antegrade use of the narrower bit.

The screw length is selected by measuring with a ruler the length from mid P-2 to the tip of the fingertip, and then subtracting 4 mm. The screw is inserted from distal to proximal—its leading tip is seen exiting the base of P-3. The screw tip is then placed in the hole previously made in the head of P-2. The assistant compresses the coapted surfaces,

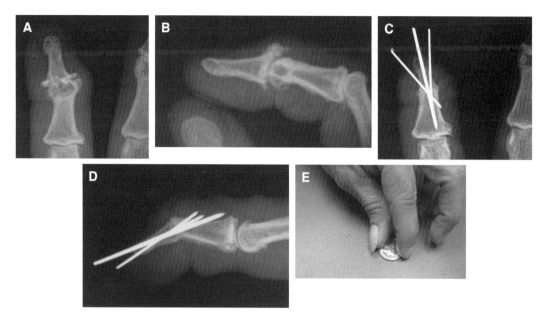

Fig. 1. DIP joint fusion with K-wires (*A*) Preoperative anteroposterior (AP) radiograph. (*B*) Preoperative lateral radiograph. (*C*) Postoperative AP radiograph. (*D*) Postoperative lateral radiograph. (*E*) Fused index DIP joint in flexion facilitates prehension.

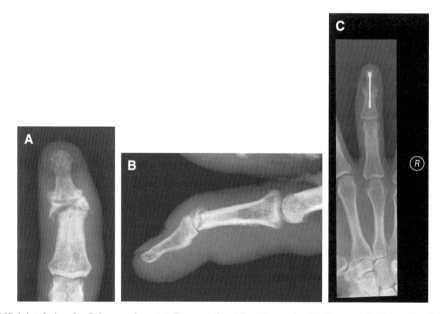

Fig. 2. DIP joint fusion for P-2 nonunion. (*A*) Preoperative AP radiograph. (*B*) Preoperative lateral radiograph. (*C*) Postoperative AP radiograph. (*D*) Postoperative lateral radiograph. (*E*) Composite flexion after DIP joint fusion. (*F*) Fused index DIP joint in extension interferes slightly with tip-to-tip prehension.

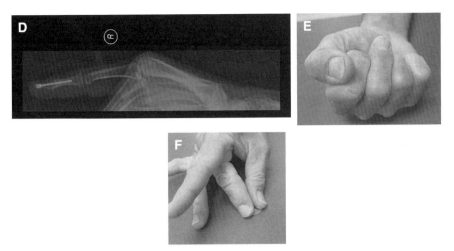

Fig. 2 (*continued*)

and the screw is inserted until it is buried beneath hyponychial skin. After an additional few turns of the screwdriver, a fluoroscopic image is taken to ensure that the head is nearly buried in P-3. At this point, additional compression is possible across the nonthreaded portion of the Herbert screw, if necessary. The extensor tendon is repaired with absorbable suture if possible, and the skin is closed. A postoperative dressing is removed at 5 to 7 days postoperatively, and motion is started. Sutures are removed between 2 and 3 weeks postoperatively.

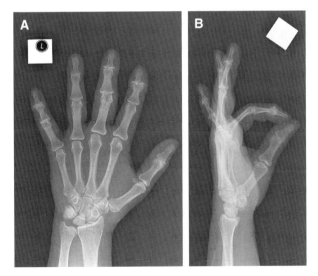

Fig. 3. DIP joint fusion for osteoarthritic index and small finger disease with concomitant long finger PIP joint implant arthroplasty. (*A*) Preoperative AP radiograph. (*B*) Preoperative lateral radiograph. (*C*) Postoperative AP radiograph. (*D*) Postoperative lateral radiograph.

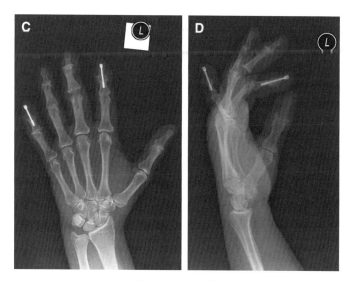

Fig. 3 (*continued*)

Summary

   Though DIP joint fusion can be successfully achieved with K-wires in both the osteoarthritic and rheumatoid patient, their use is often somewhat of an inconvenience to the patient. They prohibit showering, may become infected, may back out and catch on clothing, and surely slow down mobilization of the rest of the finger [1]. For optimal prehension, a modest amount of DIP joint flexion is required, however. Thus, one advantage of K-wires is that they allow fusion in 5° to 10° of flexion (Fig. 1). In the rheumatoid patient in particular, bone stock may be so compromised that getting enough purchase with wires alone can be challenging.

   Since making the transition to the Herbert screw, hardware-related complications and patient dissatisfaction with obligatory postoperative functional limitations until union is achieved have been eliminated. Despite the fact that the fusion must occur without flexion—a necessity to ensure intramedullary placement of the screw—patients seem to adapt well (Fig. 2). One further potential disadvantage of screw fixation is the issue of size mismatch between phalanx and screw—especially in the small finger. Though cautious insertion is justified, precise technique allows use even in the small finger—a benefit when early motion is indicated; for example, when concomitant proximal interphalangeal (PIP) implant arthroplasty is performed in an adjacent digit. This device is contraindicated, obviously, if future PIP joint arthroplasty is anticipated in the same finger (Fig. 3).

References

[1] Burton RI, Margles SW, Lunseth PA. Small-joint arthrodesis in the hand. J Hand Surg [Am] 1986;11:678–82.

[2] Stern PJ, Fulton DB. Distal interphalangeal joint arthrodesis: an analysis of complications. J Hand Surg [Am] 1992;17:1139–45.

[3] Faithfull DK, Herbert TJ. Small joint fusions of the hand using the Herbert bone screw. J Hand Surg [Br] 1984;9:167–8.

[4] El-Hadidi S, Al-Kdah H. Distal interphalangeal joint arthrodesis with Herbert screw. Hand Surg 2003;8:21–4.

[5] Wyrsch B, Dawson J, Aufranc S, et al. Distal interphalangeal joint arthrodesis comparing tension-band wire and Herbert screw: a biomechanical and dimensional analysis. J Hand Surg [Am] 1996;21:438–43.

[6] Brutus JP, Palmer AK, Mosher JF, et al. Use of a headless compressive screw for distal interphalangeal joint arthrodesis in digits: clinical outcome and review of complications. J Hand Surg [Am] 2006;31:85–9.

ELSEVIER
SAUNDERS

Hand Clin 22 (2006) 211–220

HAND
CLINICS

Thumb Metacarpophalangeal Arthritis: Arthroplasty or Fusion?

Charles S. Day, MD, MBA[a,b,*], Miguel A. Ramirez, BS[a,b]

[a]Department of Orthopaedic Surgery, Beth Israel Deaconess Medical Center, 330 Brookline Avenue,
E/CC2, Boston, MA 02215, USA
[b]Harvard Medical School, 260 Longwood Avenue, Boston, MA 02115, USA

The human thumb assumes 50% of the workload of the human hand [1], and is therefore the most important digit. As such, the thumb has a propensity for the development of osteoarthritis. Moreover, the thumb is also often diseased, in anywhere from 68% to 80% of patients who have rheumatoid arthritis (RA) [1,2].

Much attention over the years has been given to the carpalmetacarpal (CMC) joint of the thumb, whereas the metacarpophalangeal (MP) joint of the thumb remains largely unstudied. The purpose of this article is to review the etiology of thumb MP joint arthritis, and discuss the different treatment options of this condition.

Incidence and etiology

Although range of motion of the thumb MP joint in healthy individuals is only a few degrees [3,4], disease of the joint, whether due to instability or pain, can bring about significant disability and loss of function to patients [5]. Pain about this joint is usually a result of arthritis, whose etiology may be either degenerative, post-traumatic, or inflammatory—most commonly RA. Isolated degenerative arthritis of the thumb is very rare, and when seen, a specific etiology must be sought [6]. Osteoarthritis of the MCP joint is usually related to prior injury [7], whereas in the

rheumatoid thumb, it is usually a result of ligamentous and capsular involvement as well as erosion of the joint surfaces [7].

RA, which affects roughly 6% of the general population [8], is the primary cause of MP arthritis. RA is a condition that may start as an antigen-dependant activation of T-cells with an array of downstream effects, such as activation of proinflammatory cells from bone marrow and circulation, secretion of cytokines and proteases by macrophages and fibroblast-like synovial cells, active synovial tissue proliferation, and finally, autoantibody production [9]. This autoimmune type of inflammation results in the key feature that separates RA from osteo- or post-traumatic arthritis—soft-tissue damage that renders the joint unstable. As a result, treatment must be geared to not only pain relief, but also to return stability to the joint.

MP arthritis in the rheumatoid thumb typically starts with a boutonnière deformity [1,2]. Boutonnière deformity is a debilitating and painful condition whose feature is MP flexion and interphalangeal (IP) hyperextension of the thumb [1]. As part of the disease progression, active extension of the MP joint is lost as the central slip over the MP joint subluxes around the joint below its axis of rotation, eliminating the physiological pulley system to extend this joint. As a consequence, the extension force is then transmitted to the IP joint, where it hyperextends this joint. Subsequently, MP and IP joint deformity may become fixed and contracted, possibly leading to joint dislocation and destruction [1,2]. Dislocation in the rheumatoid thumb is attributed to the destruction of the supporting soft-tissue structures, such as the collateral ligaments, whose function

* Corresponding author. Department of Orthopaedic Surgery, Beth Israel Deaconess Medical Center, 330 Brookline Avenue, E/CC2, Boston, MA 02215.
E-mail address: cday1@bidmc.harvard.edu (C.S. Day).

0749-0712/06/$ - see front matter © 2006 Elsevier Inc. All rights reserved.
doi:10.1016/j.hcl.2006.02.010

hand.theclinics.com

is to provide static joint stability. In addition, articular cartilage is usually eroded as well, as a result of the rheumatoid pannus formation in the joint [10]. Therefore, when treating the rheumatoid thumb, it is paramount to address both paint and stability of the joint.

Osteoarthritis (OA) of the MP joint is a rare disease. OA in general is thought to be a multifactorial process involving biomechanical, biochemical, genetic, and metabolic factors that lead to secondary inflammation at the joint. Osteoarthritic conditions in the thumb are usually a result of a mechanical process, such as trauma or repeated microtrauma, which results in joint surface maltracking, and in combination with the release of degenerative enzymes by chondrocytes [11] it causes articular surface degeneration. The key distinction of the osteoarthritic thumb as compared with the rheumatoid thumb is that the osteoarthritic thumb is inherently stable—its collateral ligaments are generally intact. Therefore, treatment of this condition is usually geared toward pain relief only rather than stability.

Management

Nonsurgical management

Management of MP arthritis must begin in a conservative manner. Whether MP arthritis is a result of OA or inflammatory arthritis, a careful evaluation of the functional status of the patient must be performed. In patients who have OA, the goal of early management is aimed at pain relief and quick return to activities of daily living. As a result, early, nonsurgical treatment focuses primarily on lifestyle modification, nonsteroidal anti-inflammatory drugs (NSAIDS), and splinting. This form of treatment, although not necessarily curative, provides pain relief and return to activity, while slowing the progression of arthritis and buying time before invasive treatment will be necessary.

Management of the rheumatoid thumb is more challenging than the osteoarthritic thumb, and several additional factors must be considered. First, because of its relatively fast progression, treatment of RA must be initiated early and should be closely monitored as compared with OA, which usually has a more gradual progression. In one study [12], more than 80% of RA patients at 2 years showed evidence of joint space narrowing, and approximately 65% showed erosions. Second, thorough functional status of the MP joint as well as

the rest of the thumb axis must be assessed, because the degree of involvement of other joints will dictate the treatment modality. Self-report questionnaires such as the Disorders of the Shoulder and Hand (DASH), the Arthritis Impact Measurement Scale (AIMS), and the Short-form 36 (SF-36), are adequate ways to assess the functional status of patients.

Because the progression of RA is relatively abrupt, early treatment with disease-modifying antirheumatic drugs (DMARDs) is recommended. Other early forms of treatment include: (1) rest—because RA produces fatigue and subsequent difficulty in performing everyday tasks, rest can be beneficial in reducing inflammation; (2) exercise—pain and swelling causes patients to stop using the joint, which leads to stiffness and loss of motion—by exercising, patients are able to maintain their range of motion and avoid stiffness, while strengthening the musculature, thereby providing better stability for the thumb; (3) physical therapy/occupational therapy—goals of PT and OT are not only to reduce pain and improve function, but in the case of OT, to educate the patient on joint protection and usage of assistive devices that will prolong the necessity to undergo corrective surgery [9].

Splinting provides immobilization of the involved joints, allowing for a reduction of inflammation and subsequent pain relief. Splinting may bring about temporary reduction of pain and return of function, while buying time before more invasive procedures are necessary.

When conservative treatment is unable to provide pain relief or the ability to return to activities of daily living, surgery is recommended.

Surgical treatment

Many surgical methods have been used over the years to treat MP arthritis of the thumb. The techniques implemented are dictated by the location and severity of the underlying joint pathology. Joint fusion has been the treatment of choice over the last 50 years for end-stage thumb MP osteoarthritis. In the rheumatoid thumb, the treatments of choice have been synovectomy and reconstruction of extensor apparatus as a primary treatment of mild-to-moderate joint pathology, whereas arthrodesis is the gold standard in the setting of extensive monoarticular disruption [10]. When significant pathology exists in the other joints around the thumb axis, other treatment modalities have been proposed. Thumb arthroplasty, as pioneered by Brannon and Klein in 1959 [13,14], has brought a new form of treatment for patients who have considerable thumb arthritis extending beyond the MP joint.

Whether it is arthroplasty or arthrodesis that is considered for the MP joint, surgical treatment is aimed at four goals: (1) pain relief, (2) restoring function, (3) preventing further damage, and (4) providing cosmetic improvement [7,15,16]. In the case of the unstable rheumatoid thumb, surgical treatment is also aimed at correcting the instability about this joint.

Arthroplasty

Arthroplasty of the MP joint is a useful technique in the attempt to maintain thumb length, relieve stress about the CMC joint, and improve positioning of the thumb tip [15]. Arthroplasty of the MP joint of the thumb is relatively easy to accomplish, because the MP joint anatomy approximates that of a simple hinge [15].

Brannon and Klein reported the first prosthetic MP joint in 1959 [13]. This early prosthesis was a hinged replica of the MP joint, first constructed of stainless steel and then titanium [13]. Many problems were reported with this device. Out of 12 subjects tested, 2 patients developed deformity because of prosthesis migration into the proximal phalanx. In 2 other patients, a screw at the hinge portion became loose and needed to be tightened. These unsatisfactory results and high number of complications sparked the search for better methods of arthroplasty, and since then various materials and techniques have been developed, such as Swanson's silicone arthroplasty and the hinged metal-polyethylene arthroplasty.

The primary indications for arthroplasty are considerable arthridities in which there appears to be significant involvement of the IP or CMC joint [7,14,15]. It is important to note that most rheumatoid patients are able to accommodate to level of normal activities of daily living, even at the presence of gross clinical deformity. Therefore, it is only in the patient who complains of significant persistent pain caused by destruction of the MP joint that arthroplasty should be considered [14].

Swanson silicone arthroplasty

Silicone rubber prostheses were first introduced in the 1960s by Swanson [7,8]. The need for a material such as silicone arose, as Swanson stated, from the observation that metal implants

at that time were shown to be primarily ineffective and had minimal acceptance. Moreover, these implants were shown to corrode after some time, and the bone was unable to tolerate the metal [8,13]. The idea for the use of silicone by Swanson in his prosthesis came from the observed success of intramedullary stemmed silicone rubber implants to cushion the end of long bones after lower extremity amputations. This provided a framework for an inert, flexible, and lightweight alternative to the conventional titanium or stainless steel prostheses.

The material chosen by Swanson and coworkers was Silastic, a silicone dioxide elastomer created by the Dow Corning Corp of Midland, Michigan [7,8]. Swanson made this his material of choice because it is inert, stable at high temperature, and it is very durable [8,14]. In the original report [8], it was stated that this material could withstand greater than 50 million repetitions without failure. The feature of the Swanson arthroplasty that sets it apart from other types of arthroplasties is that this implant is not a total joint replacement, but rather a noncemented spacer between the metacarpal and proximal phalanx (Fig. 1). As a result of this, instability is of

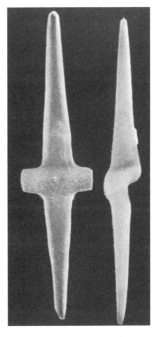

Fig. 1. Original Swason Silastic MP joint spacer. (*From* Swanson AB. Silicone rubber implants for replacement of arthritic or destroyed joints in the hand. Surg Clin North Am 1968;48(5):1117; with permission.)

concern, and therefore, adequate reconstruction of the collateral ligaments is paramount.

The surgical technique involves a dorsal incision over the MP joint, with dissection carried down through the subcutaneous tissue until the extensor hoods are exposed [8]. The extensor hood is dislocated ulnarly and the fibers are carefully dissected away from the synovium. A thorough synovectomy is performed, and if there is considerable joint surface ablation, the metacarpal head may be osteotomized. The ulnar and radial collateral ligaments are released and then tagged with 2-0 nonabsorbable suture for future attachment [14]. In RA patients, the collateral ligaments often demonstrate some compromise in their integrity; however, any soft tissue around the ligament may be tagged as part of the reconstruction later. Once ligament/soft-tissue tagging is accomplished, the intramedullary canal of the metacarpal and the proximal phalanx are reamed with the aid of a curette or a broach. The implant is subsequently inserted on the proximal end first, and then the distal end is flexed and guided into the proximal phalanx intramedullary canal. The collateral ligaments or any of the surrounding capsular tissue are then reattached to their anatomical position for stability of the joint. Extensor pollicis brevis (EPB) tendon is subsequently sutured to the proximal phalanx (Fig. 2A). The medial and lateral expansions are sutured over the EPB (Fig. 2B), restoring the intrinsic mechanism. Finally, the EPB tendon is pulled distally and sutured in the midline over the MP joint (Fig. 2C). Pulling the tendon distally and anchoring its proximal end relaxes its distal insertion on the distal phalanx, thus relieving extension force over the IP joint [17]. Once this is complete, the wound is copiously irrigated and closed.

Following Swanson's original report on his new prosthesis, Swanson and Herndon [17] reviewed 42 rheumatoid thumbs that had undergone arthroplasty with the Swanson spacer. Follow-up was 2 to 6.5 years. Forty-two of the patients (100%) reported positive results, described as a resolution of their pain. The study authors also reported that 6 individuals who received arthroplasty had previously received arthrodesis in the opposite thumb. Out of these 6 individuals, 5 reported that their arthroplasty thumb felt better than their fused thumb, and the remaining patient said that he could tell no difference between them. More recent studies have also shown great success from this type of arthroplasty. A 1990 study [18] also showed good results from the

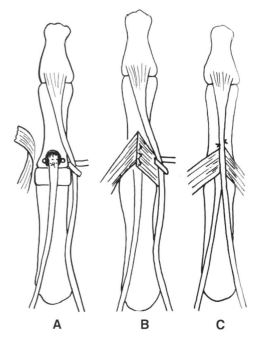

Fig. 2. (A) Once implant has been inserted, EPB tendon is reattached to the proximal phalanx. (B) Medial and lateral expansions are sutured over the EPB tendon. (C) Extensor pollicis longus tendon is pulled distally and sutured to the midline over the MP joint. Pulling the tendon distally and tacking it to the extensor mechanism releases pressure on the distal end, thus releasing flexion restraint from distal phalanx. (From Swanson AB, Herndon JH. Flexible (silicone) implant arthroplasty of the metacarpophalangeal joint of the thumb. J Bone Joint Surg Am 1977;59(3):364; with permission from the Journal of Bone and Joint Surgery, Inc.)

Swanson thumb MP prosthesis. Forty-three thumbs were looked at in rheumatoid patients. The average range of active motion was reported at 25°, with a flexion arc from 15° to 40°. Forty of these patients (93%) had improvements in activities of daily living. Only one thumb required reoperation with arthrodesis. Moreover, the authors report that only 3 patients showed disease progression radiographically—1 at the IP joint, and 2 at the CMC.

Not all investigators report such great outcomes from the Swanson Silastic prosthesis, however. In a 1975 study out of Sweden [19], the investigators decided to study the Swanson prosthesis radiographically on a variety of fingers of patients who had RA, in an effort to determine the integrity and the durability of 104 Silastic implants. The investigators found radiographic evidence of prosthesis failure in many asymptomatic patients. They went on to describe three types of failure of the prosthesis: (1) surface damage (2 of 42), (2) cracking or fragmentation of midsection (14 of 104) (Fig. 3), and (3) stem fracture (11 of 104). Overall, 25% of prostheses failed within 1.5 to 5.5 years. As for the causes of failure of the implant, the study authors attributed them to several different reasons: (1) deformation of implant—this was described as a "pinch," which was a sharp, palmarly bend of the implant at the junction of the distal stem and midsection; (2) laceration of the implant surface—because of the nature of the polymer, any laceration of the surface led to a cracking of the device; (3) lipid absorption—body fluids were absorbed by the silicon dioxide, weakening the polymer [19]. From the study results, it was clear that these prostheses failed at a much higher rate than had been reported previously, and because many of these failures were not clinically evident, further studies needed to take place with long enough follow-up to make these failures clinically apparent.

Two other studies [20,21] have also shown that the Silastic material is prone to fracture, although these clinical studies did not involve the thumb. Bass and colleagues [20] reported an implant failure rate of 45%, whereas Lourie [22] found an implant failure rate of 27.5%. More surprisingly, both studies reported high patient satisfaction

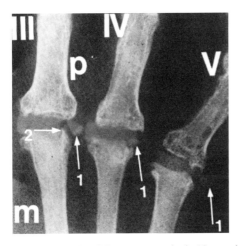

Fig. 3. Radiograph of Swanson prosthesis 12 months postoperatively at MP joints III, IV, and V, showing two different types of implant failure: (1) fragmentation of implant; (2) sharp bone edge on metacarpal bone. m, metacarpal bone; p, proximal phalanx. (*From* Hagert CG, Eiken O, Ohlsson NM, et al. Metacarpophalangeal joint implants. I. Roentgenographic study on the Silastic finger joint implant, Swanson design. Scand J Plast Reconstr Surg 1975,9(2):152; with permission.)

despite the high failure rate. Bass and colleagues showed that fracture of the implant was not related to patient satisfaction and 80% would undergo the procedure again [20], whereas Schmidt and colleagues [21] showed relief of pain in 75% of patients.

These studies show that despite the relatively high fracture rate, the Swanson prosthesis works relatively well for patients in terms of pain relief and return to activity. Based on these results, the authors extrapolate that the implant fracture rate in the thumb must also be relatively high, but as the other studies also show, these implant failures may not translate into clinical failures.

Hinged metal-polyethylene arthroplasty

Although shown to be successful, the Swanson arthroplasty was not a recreation of the MP joint. The Swanson arthroplasty was more of an elastic spacer whose flexibility allowed for much play at the joint interface. As an attempt to anatomically recreate the MP joint in the style of Brannon in the 1950s [13], Steffee [23] designed a hinged metal-and-polyethylene device in 1973 that would approximate a total joint reconstruction similar to that performed in the knee and hip. This new procedure was designed to provide more anatomical stability than the Swanson spacer by its hinged design, which approximated the normal MP joint architecture and restricted the amount of dynamic freedom at the joint interface. The polyethylene proximal part was designed with a dorsally displaced stem to bring down the center of rotation of the joint to the inferior portion of the metacarpal head [23]. The distal metal component snap-locks into the proximal component, providing a tight hinge at the joint interface. The volar lip was also designed to block flexion beyond 40° in an effort to prevent flexion deformity if the extensor mechanism subluxes (Fig. 4).

In 1981, Beckenbaugh and Steffee published a report evaluating 42 prosthetic replacements in the thumbs of 38 patients [23]. Of the 42 procedures, 33 were performed for rheumatic disease, 8 for degenerative or traumatic osteoarthritis, and the remaining case was a revision. In this cohort of patients, postoperative range of motion averaged -12° extension to 28° flexion, for an average motion arc of 16°. Pain was reported absent in 100% of patients, and no infections of fractures were reported in the follow-up period. The report authors, however, described the results of this prosthesis as "disappointing" because of the

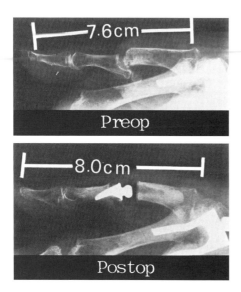

Fig. 4. Radiograph before (*top*) and after surgery (*bottom*) with Steffee prosthesis. Measurements show an increase of 0.4 cm in thumb length. (*From* Beckenbaugh RB, Steffee AD. Total joint arthroplasty for the metacarpophalangeal joint of the thumb—a preliminary report. Orthopedics 1981;4(3):297; with permission.)

very shallow 16° motion arc. Functionally and esthetically, there was no objective difference between thumbs with fusion and thumbs with this type of arthroplasty. Moreover, Beckenbaugh and Steffee proposed that although the complication rate was minimal, it could be potentially higher than that reported in this study for the surgeon that is not as well-versed with the implant technique [23].

In 1994, a newer metal-polyethylene implant was created by Harris and Dias [24] in efforts to address the relatively low motion arc attained with the Steffee prosthesis. This particular implant was designed similarly to the Steffee total joint implant, made from cobalt chrome molybdenum alloy and ultra-high-density polyethylene. The joint surface was determined from cadaveric specimens and MRI images from several adult patients. Unique to this design were uncemented finned polyethylene plugs, which allowed metacarpal component motion, hopefully giving more mobility about the MP joint.

This implant was reviewed by Harris and Dias in 2003 [24]. In this study, 13 joints in eight patients were replaced and followed over 5 years. From this cohort, the investigators reported no implant failures. Out of the 13 implants, they reported one infection that required revision at 3 months, 2 joints

that showed lucency in the area around the phalangeal component, and 1 joint that showed a 2-mm subsidence of the metacarpal component. Seven of the eight patients were pain-free, and the remaining patient had minor discomfort. Moreover, Harris and Dias reported a joint movement arc improvement from 27° to 60° and improvement on a validated Patient Evaluated Measure (PEM) questionnaire from 77% to 9% [24].

Arthrodesis

For years, arthrodesis has been the gold standard in treating isolated end-stage MP arthritis, whether inflammatory or post-traumatic arthropathies [25]. Arthrodesis is able to provide effective pain relief as well as restore stability to the joint, even in the setting of severe arthritis. [1,3,7,10,25]. The key to why MP fusion in the thumb is so successful lies in the relatively negligible loss of motion that results from MP fusion. The functional goal of the thumb is to be able to oppose to at least the ring finger, or preferably the small finger. Because the CMC joint of the thumb has many degrees of freedom, even with a fused MP joint, patients are still able to oppose the tip of the thumb to the tip of the ring or small finger; thus fusion of the MP joint is able to eliminate pain, while affecting thumb biomechanics at a minimal level.

The goal of arthrodesis is to be able to allow union at a biomechanically functional position for the patient [26]. Several authors estimate this position to be roughly 15° of flexion, whereas minimal variation exists in the recommendation of both internal/external rotation and radial/ulnar deviation. By establishing fusion at the MP joint, the surgeon is also able to potentially save involvement of other joints of the thumb [25]. For example, by fusing the MP joint between 20° and 40° of flexion, stress can be relieved from the CMC joint by minimizing the activity required at the CMC for thumb opposition. This position not only provides better pain relief in patients who have an already arthritic CMC, but also protects it from worsening arthritis [25].

Many MP arthrodesis techniques have been described [1,3,5,10,16,22,26]. All procedures, however, can be divided into two key components: (1) metacarpal/proximal phalanx osteotomy, and (2) bone fixation. In joint fusion, there are two main types of osteotomies currently used: (1) a flat cut at the desired angle of fusion, and (2) the shallow V or "chevron" osteotomy. The

latter type allows both bone fragments to fit together, preventing them from sliding from the
position of fixation, but it needs more precision
cuts to accomplish the desired angle. Both types
of osteotomies work relatively equally, so the
type of osteotomy performed usually depends on
the surgeon's preference.

Numerous methods of fixation have been performed over the years, ranging from Kirschner-
wire to cannulated screw fixation. The technique
described by Omer [27] in 1968 is the most widely
used [3]. In this procedure, a posterior approach
to the joint is established, and the extensor mechanism is divided at the MP joint, with consequent
release of the collateral ligaments from the metacarpal [27]. After appropriate exposure of the joint
is obtained, the joint surfaces of the metacarpal and
proximal phalanx are osteotomized to generate
a chevron-shaped mortise (Fig. 5) with the point
oriented proximally. This osteotomy allows for
the placement of the joint at the desired angle.
Once both surfaces are opposed and desired functional orientation is acquired, stabilization is
achieved by the placement of Kirschner wires to
hold fixation. Soft-tissue release of thumb web is
done whenever necessary [3].

This procedure has been relatively successful.
Stanley and colleagues [3] studied 42 arthrodeses

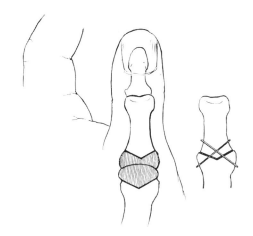

Fig. 5. Chevron osteotomy as described by Omer in 1968.
Metacarpal and proximal phalanx are cut in a shallow V
fashion. Metacarpal is inclined volarly to give desired angle of fusion. Once the two bones are approximated, fixation is accomplished by placement of two crossing
Kirschner wires. (*From* Omer GE Jr. Evaluation and reconstruction of the forearm and hand after acute traumatic peripheral nerve injuries. J Bone Joint Surg Am
1968;50(7):1469; with permission from the Journal of
Bone and Joint Surgery, Inc.)

with the Omer technique, and followed up for an
average of 22.5 months postoperatively. Eighty-
three percent of fusions were reported as successful in pain reduction and return to activity. Mean
angle of fusion was 11.5° of flexion. The main indication for arthrodesis reported in this study was
pain. In 36% of hands reviewed, MP arthrodesis
was supplemented by other procedures. There
were five nonunions (12%). The angle of fusion,
which ranged from 0° to 20° flexion, was shown
not to correlate with the patient's ability to oppose the thumb, nor was it related to the amount
of pain reported in the postoperative follow-up.
Two major complications were reported from
this procedure. Both were extensor pollicis longus
(EPL) tendon ruptures as a result of longitudinal
wires placed during fixation.

The observation that compression at a fracture
or osteotomy site helps achieve union served as
the basis for the introduction of tension band
arthrodesis. In the finger, the power of the flexors
far exceeds that of the extensors [28]. Tension
band arthrodesis uses this concept to turn the
force of flexion into a force of interfragmentary
compression, and thus aid the process of union
(Fig. 6). The added benefit of this procedure
over conventional Kirschner-wire fixation is its
ability to provide compression of bone opposition
at the osteotomy site and relieve stiffness from
other joints by allowing early movement [26].

Feldon and coworkers [25] and Inglis and
Hamlin [10] advocate for fusion at 15° flexion,
15° abduction, and 15° internal rotation. They
also stress that this not a fixed rule, because the
other joints must also be taken into consideration.
For example, if the CMC joint contains significant
pathology, MP joint should be fused in more flexion, as much as 25° [25]. Increased flexion at the
MP joint when the CMC is compromised allows
the thumb tip to approximate the ring or small
finger. If CMC is diseased and MP joint is fused
at too shallow of an angle, thumb opposition
will be compromised and subsequent discomfort
and disability will ensue.

Tension band has been shown to be more
effective than conventional Kirschner-wire fusion
of the MCP joint alone [10,26]. In one study [26],
203 MP and IP arthrodesis were reviewed comparing tension-band to Kirschner-wire only fixation.
Infection rates were found to be much higher in
the Kirschner-wire than in the tension-band group
(18% versus 2% respectively). Of these infections
in the Kirschner-wire group, 42% lead to a nonunion at the MCP joint. Rearthrodesis rates for

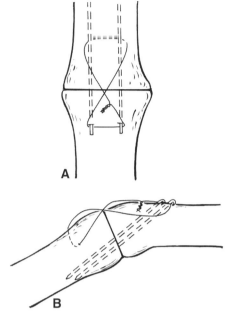

Fig. 6. Tension band technique. (*A*) Dorsal view. (*B*) Lateral view. (*From* I Jsselstein CB, van Egmond DB, Hovius SE, et al. Results of small-joint arthrodesis: comparison of Kirschner wire fixation with tension band wire technique. J Hand Surg [Am] 1992;17(5):953; with permission.)

over the guide wire and a 3.0-mm screw is then secured (Fig. 7).

One study in 2004 [5] looked at the cannulated screw procedure in 26 patients. Their indications for surgery were instability, chronic instability, inflammatory arthritis, and fixed boutonnière. Twenty-five of 26 patients achieved both clinical and radiographic fusion, and reported pain relief as well as return to daily activities. Average time to union was 10 weeks, with a mean fusion angle of 18°. At an average of 32 months, (range 21–44 months) there was one nonunion that was achieved fusion via tension band. There were no reported infections or need for removal of hardware.

Discussion

MP arthritis of the thumb is a potentially debilitating disorder whose treatment is relative successful for the surgeon who thoroughly evaluates the entire thumb axis, because involvement of other joints will dictate the most appropriate treatment.

Fusion is generally successful, and very little variability in results exists between methods. This treatment option is also supported by most of the existing literature on this topic [5,7,12,14]. Osteotomy type, whether flat or chevron, makes no

the tension-band group were also shown to be lower than the Kirschner-wire group (5% versus 15%). In essence, Kirschner-wire MP arthrodesis was successful 85% of the time, whereas the tension-band procedure had a success rate of 95%. The major drawback to tension-band arthrodesis is that this procedure can be technically challenging and time-consuming.

Arthrodesis of the MP joint using a cannulated screw and threaded washer has been reported [5] as an easier way to provide compression at the osteotomy site and improve union rates. In this procedure, performed under regional anesthesia, the extensor mechanism and the joint capsule are divided at the interval between the EPB and the EPL tendons. A chevron osteotomy is then performed, followed by bone segment approximation. The thumb is placed at key pinch configuration with 10° to 15° of flexion, neutral rotation, and radial/ulnar deviation [5]. A 1.1-mm threaded guide pin is passed from the dorsal aspect of the metacarpal through the metacarpal head, and into the medullary canal of the phalanx. Once this is complete, a threaded washer is placed

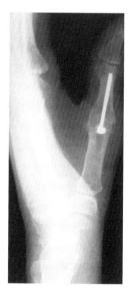

Fig. 7. Anteroposterior (AP) radiograph showing MP fusion using a cannulated screw and washer. (*From* Schmidt CC, Zimmer SM, Boles SD. Arthrodesis of the thumb metacarpophalangeal joint using a cannulated screw and threaded washer. J Hand Surg [Am] 2004; 29(6):1048; with permission.)

significant difference in overall fusion rate. Compression across the osteotomy site has been shown to promote better fusion. In the past, tension banding was the best way to provide compression across the osteotomy site. The drawback to this procedure was is that it is technically challenging and time-consuming. Technological advancement in fixation hardware has brought on several new types of cannulated headless screws that allow for easy and fast compression. These screws provide all of the benefits of tension banding in a fraction of the time. Results of these compression screws are very similar to tension banding, and this is the authors' preferred method of fixation.

Arthroplasty remains a viable option in patients who have significant CMC or IP joint involvement. Patients who find the most benefit from this procedure are those who have significant CMC involvement, such that opposition of the thumb is very painful. In these patients, the extra motion over the MP joint relieves pressure at the CMC, and therefore reduces pain on active use of the hand.

Overall, the authors recommend fusion as a first option for the rheumatoid or osteoarthritic patient who has monoarticular involvement of the MP joint of the thumb, because this procedure is relatively simple, provides good pain relief, and does not significantly limit range of motion of the thumb axis. In patients who have extensive involvement of the CMC or the IP joint, the authors recommend arthroplasty as an effective way to remove strain at these joints, prevent further injury, and relieve pain. When it comes to choosing between Silastic or metal-polyethylene implants, the authors do not have much experience with the metal-polyethylene prostheses, and the data are still scarce in demonstrating any improvement over the Swanson prosthesis. Although it has been shown to have a high fracture rate, the Swanson Silastic arthroplasty has been used for a much longer period of time, and has had clinical studies demonstrating 90% improvement in function. It has been the authors' experience that these fractures do not translate into clinical failures, and as a result, we therefore recommend the Swanson arthroplasty as the implant of choice when considering arthroplasty of the MP joint of the thumb.

References

[1] Terrono A, Millender L. Surgical treatment of the boutonnière rheumatoid thumb deformity. Hand Clin 1989;5(2):239–48.

[2] Manueddu CA, Bogoch ER, Hastings DE. Restoration of metacarpophalangeal extension of the thumb in inflammatory arthritis. J Hand Surg [Br] 1996; 21(5):633–9

[3] Stanley JK, Smith EJ, Muirhead AG. Arthrodesis of the metacarpo-phalangeal joint of the thumb: a review of 42 cases. J Hand Surg [Br] 1989;14(3):291–3.

[4] Yoshida R, House HO, Patterson RM, et al. Motion and morphology of the thumb metacarpophalangeal joint. J Hand Surg [Am] 2003;28(5):753–7.

[5] Schmidt CC, Zimmer SM, Boles SD. Arthrodesis of the thumb metacarpophalangeal joint using a cannulated screw and threaded washer. J Hand Surg [Am] 2004;29(6):1044–50.

[6] Feldon P, Belsky MR. Degenerative diseases of the metacarpophalangeal joints. Hand Clin 1987;3(3): 429–47.

[7] Ring D, Herndon JH. Implant arthroplasty of the metacarpophalangeal joint of the thumb. Hand Clin 2001;17(2):271–3.

[8] Swanson AB. Silicone rubber implants for replacement of arthritis or destroyed joints in the hand. Surg Clin North Am 1968;48(5):1113–27.

[9] Harris ED, Schur PH. Pathogenesis of rheumatoid arthritis. In up-to-date 2005. Available at: http://utdol.com/utd/content/topic.do?topickey=rheumart/7051&type=A&SelectedTitle=19~216. Accessed December 11, 2005.

[10] Inglis AE, Hamlin C, Sengelmann RP, et al. Reconstruction of the metacarpophalangeal joint of the thumb in rheumatoid arthritis. J Bone Joint Surg Am 1972;54(4):704–12.

[11] Mankin HJ, Brandt KD. Biochemistry and metabolism of articular cartilage in osteoarthritis. In: Moskowitz RW, Howell DS, Goldberg VC, et al, editors. Osteoarthritis: diagnosis and management. 2nd edition. Philadelphia: WB Saunders; 1992. p. 109–54.

[12] Fuchs HA, Kaye JJ, Callahan LF, et al. Evidence of significant radiographic damage in rheumatoid arthritis within the first 2 years of disease. J Rheumatol 1989;16(5):585–91.

[13] Brannon EW, Klein G. Experiences with a finger-joint prosthesis. J Bone Joint Surg Am 1959;41-A(1):87–102.

[14] Murray PM. Current status of metacarpophalangeal arthroplasty and basilar joint arthroplasty of the thumb. Clin Plast Surg 1996;23(3):395–406.

[15] Berger RA, Beckenbaugh RD, Linscheid RL. Arthroplasty in the hand and wrist. In: Green DP, Hotchkiss RN, Pederson WC, editors. Green's operative hand surgery. 4th edition. Philadelphia: Churchill Livingstone; 1999. p. 162–91.

[16] O'Brien ET. Surgical principles and planning for the rheumatoid hand and wrist. Clin Plast Surg 1996; 23(3):407–20.

[17] Swanson AB, Herndon JH. Flexible (silicone) implant arthroplasty of the metacarpophalangeal joint of the thumb. J Bone Joint Surg Am 1977;59(3): 362–8.

[18] Figgie MP, Inglis AE, Sobel M, et al. Metacarpal-phalangeal joint arthroplasty of the rheumatoid thumb. J Hand Surg [Am] 1990;15(2):210–6.

[19] Hagert CG, Eiken Ö, Ohlsson NM, et al. Metacarpophalangeal joint implants. I. Roentgenographic study on the Silastic finger joint implant, Swanson design. Scand J Plast Reconstr Surg 1975;9(2):147–57.

[20] Bass RL, Stern PJ, Nairus JG. High implant fracture incidence with Sutter silicone metacarpophalangeal joint arthroplasty. J Hand Surg [Am] 1996;21(5):813–8.

[21] Schmidt K, Miehlke RK, Witt K. Status of the endoprosthesis in rheumatic metacarpophalangeal joints. Long-term results of metacarpophalangeal prostheses using Swanson's Silastic spacers. Handchir Mikrochir Plast Chir 1996;28(5):254–64.

[22] Lourie GM. The role and implementation of metacarpophalangeal joint fusion and capsulodesis: indications and treatment alternatives. Hand Clin 2001; 17(2):255–60.

[23] Beckenbaugh RB, Steffee AD. Total joint arthroplasty for the metacarpophalangeal joint of the thumb—a preliminary report. Orthopedics 1981; 4(3):295–7.

[24] Harris D, Dias JJ. Five year results of a new total replacement prosthesis for the finger metacarpophalangeal joints. J Hand Surg [Br] 2003;28(5):432–8.

[25] Feldon P, Terrono AL, Nalebuff EA, et al. Rheumatoid arthritis and other connective tissue diseases. In: Green DP, Hotchkiss RN, Pederson WC, editors. Green's operative hand surgery. 4th edition. Philadelphia: Churchill Livingstone; 1999. p. 1726–39.

[26] I Jsselstein CB, van Egmond DB, Hovius SE, et al. Results of small-joint arthrodesis: comparison of Kirschner wire fixation with tension band wire technique. J Hand Surg [Am] 1992;17(5):952–6.

[27] Omer GE Jr. Evaluation and reconstruction of the forearm and hand after acute traumatic peripheral nerve injuries. J Bone Joint Surg Am 1968;50(7): 1454–78.

[28] Allende BT, Engelem JC. Tension-band arthrodesis in the finger joints. J Hand Surg [Am] 1980;5(3): 269–71.

Degenerative and Post-Traumatic Arthritis Affecting the Carpometacarpal Joints of the Fingers

Thomas R. Hunt III, MD

Division of Orthopaedic Surgery, The University of Alabama, Birmingham School of Medicine,
930 Faculty Office Tower, 510 20th Street South, Birmingham, AL 35294-3409, USA

CMC joint fractures and fracture/dislocations involving the fingers are relatively common injuries that infrequently result in chronic disability. Persistent pain and dysfunction, usually manifesting as diminished grip strength, typically result from late instability and secondary joint degeneration from missed or maltreated fourth and fifth CMC joint injuries, or from multiple CMC joint fracture/dislocations caused by high energy trauma. As is the case with Bennett's fractures, symptomatic post-traumatic arthritis involving the small finger CMC joint is less frequent than might otherwise be expected, perhaps because of the relatively unconstrained nature of both joints [1]. The laxity may confer a certain degree of protection in the post-traumatic state. Similarly, degenerative joint changes manifesting as metacarpal bosses are infrequently symptomatic, and when present, rarely necessitate surgical treatment. This article reviews the relevant anatomy and epidemiology, and details treatment algorithms for symptomatic patients who have degenerative and post-traumatic problems affecting the finger CMC joints.

Anatomy, pathomechanics, and epidemiology

The finger carpometacarpal joints define the fixed unit of the hand, serving as the base for digital mobility. Stability is conferred primarily thorough the extensive ligamentous labyrinth [2].

The second and third CMC joints are highly constrained by the ligamentous anatomy as well as by the joint contours. In addition to other articulations, the second metacarpal base keys into the trapezium as an inverted "V," and the third metacarpal base keys into the capitate, often with a dorsoradial proximal projection providing a degree of added stability. Allowed motion in these joints is less than 5° [3]. Progressively more mobility is noted ulnarly. Most authors estimate a 15° flexion/extension arc for the fourth CMC joint and a 30° arc for the fifth CMC joint. The articular anatomy of the fifth CMC joint is variable, but generally resembles that seen in the trapeziometacarpal joint of the thumb with a concave (volar/dorsal) hamate facet and a correspondingly convex metacarpal base. This shallow, concavoconvex "saddle joint" allows for flexion/extension, rotation, and translation [4], facilitating cupping and flattening of the palm as well as opposition of the fifth ray.

The most frequent injuries, fractures of the fourth and fifth metacarpal bases with or without dorsal dislocation, result from striking a solid object with a clenched fist in the majority of cases, and a direct blow to the area in a minority of cases [5]. Yoshida and colleagues [6] duplicated the pathomechanics of a closed fist blow using a cadaver model, and found that specific patterns of injury were dependent on direction and degree of applied force, position of the joint, and ligamentous constraints. Plain radiographs significantly underestimated the extent and complexity of the injury produced. Kjaer-Petersen and coworkers [7] reported on their treatment of 64 intra-articular fifth metacarpal base fractures using both closed and open techniques. The majority

The author is a consultant to the Arthrotek/Biomet Corporation and an education consultant for Stryker Corporation.

E-mail address: Thomas.Hunt@ortho.uab.edu

of the fractures included the commonly observed volar radial fragment held reduced to the fourth metacarpal base via strong intermetacarpal liga ments. They improved the intra-articular reduc tion in fewer than 55% of patients despite "relatively easy" elimination of subluxation. Not only is it difficult to appreciate the full spectrum of injury radiographically, but reduction and sta bilization of the fragments may be problematic.

Despite relative consensus regarding the path omechanics, resulting pathoanatomy, and the re quirement for correction of joint subluxation, authors disagree on the need for anatomic joint restoration and the long-term impact of articular incongruity on patient outcome and even on radiographic endpoints. Lundeen and Shin [8] ret rospectively reviewed 22 patients who had isolated intra-articular fractures of the base of the fifth metacarpal at an average of 43 months following injury. All fractures were treated by closed reduc tion and cast immobilization. Twenty patients reported good or excellent results despite radiographic evidence of mild arthrosis in 9. Out come was independent of specific fracture pattern, degree of subluxation, or intra-articular incongru ity and arthrosis, as judged using plain radio graphs. Kjaer-Petersen and colleagues [7] also found that quality of the reduction did not seem to directly influence outcome, and the result was not impacted by the presence of arthrosis at me dian follow-up time of 4.3 years; however, 39% of their patients sampled by questionnaire com plained of intermittent pain with gripping, and 49% of their patients examined demonstrated de creased grip strength. Bora and Didizian [9] tied outcome to fracture displacement. One of 7 pa tients who had displaced fractures in their series re quired arthrodesis. Decreased grip strength was the most common disabling symptom.

Despite some studies indicating a high fre quency of symptoms following these common injuries, most surgeons rarely see patients who have significant chronic complaints after adequate initial treatment of CMC fracture/dislocations. The need for surgical treatment in this population of patients is even less common. Pellegrini [10] hy pothesized that in the case of Bennett's fractures, normal joint surface incongruity and infrequent contact of the metacarpal's displaced articular sur face with the remainder of the joint may exert a protective effect over late post-traumatic sequelae of residual articular fracture deformity. This same concept may be applicable to fifth CMC joint injuries, so called "reverse Bennett's fractures."

Degenerative arthritis involving the finger CMC joints usually presents as a dorsal carpo metacarpal boss projecting from the radial third metacarpal base or the ulnar second metacarpal base, often involving the capitate, and accompa nied by a ganglion cyst in 30% of cases [11]. The hypertrophic bony spurs are thought to result from repetitive forces acting on these two rigid joints that serve as the stable pillars of the hand. Fusi and colleagues [12] obtained a history of di rect trauma to the region in 24% of their operated patients. Carpometacarpal bosses are equally common in men and women. These patients typi cally present for treatment in their 20s and 30s [12], though significant symptoms related to these hypertrophic changes are uncommon.

Treatment of post-traumatic arthrosis

Patients who present with symptomatic post traumatic CMC arthrosis generally complain of pain over the involved joint aggravated by grip ping, shaking hands, and occupation-specific or sports-specific activities. A percentage of these patients present simply to determine the cause for their intermittent discomfort, but a number of others have daily, bothersome complaints. Fre quently subtle instability is present on examina tion and may be a significant contributing factor.

First line treatment is nonoperative for this population of patients. It involves education, activity modification, local treatment with ice, intermittent splinting, and use of nonsteroidal anti-inflammatory drugs (NSAIDs). Because these joints are often quite narrowed and difficult to inject, cortisone is rarely employed. Patients who have frequent and disabling symptoms require surgical intervention. The most common and accepted surgical treatment is arthrodesis; how ever, in specific cases of fifth CMC joint arthritis, some surgeons have successfully used resection arthroplasty [13], silicone implant arthroplasty [14], tendon interposition arthroplasty [15], and arthroscopic assessment followed by limited open joint debridement.

Gainor and coworkers [15] reviewed their expe rience in eight patients who underwent interposi tional arthroplasty for treatment of fifth CMC joint post-traumatic arthritis. A limited resection of either the metacarpal base or distal hamate was performed, followed by interposition of palmaris longus, repair of the dorsal carpometacarpal liga ment, and temporary joint pinning. At an average

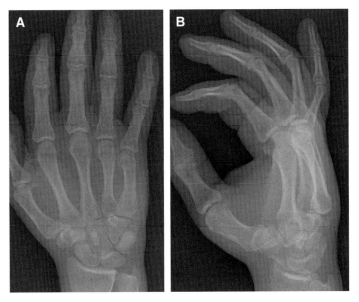

Fig. 1. (*A*) Anteroposterior (AP) and (*B*) lateral radiographs depicting a missed fifth CMC joint fracture/dislocation 4 months postinjury.

final follow-up of 5 years, there was no evidence of instability. Net increase in grip strength averaged 30%. All patients rated their functional result and cosmetic appearance as good or excellent despite an average 4 mm loss of length of the fifth ray. Radiographs revealed "egg cup" remodeling or metaphyseal hypertrophy.

This author has used a 0.8 mm investigational arthroscope (InnerVue, Arthrotek, Biomet Corporation, Warsaw, Indiana) to evaluate the fifth CMC joint and to direct limited open debridement of the joint in select athletes who have mild arthritic changes unresponsive to conservative management. This intervention has provided effective short- and medium-term relief of symptoms, and has allowed virtually uninterrupted sports participation. It is likely that as arthroscopic instrumentation improves and techniques evolve, this approach will find its place in the hand surgeon's armamentarium.

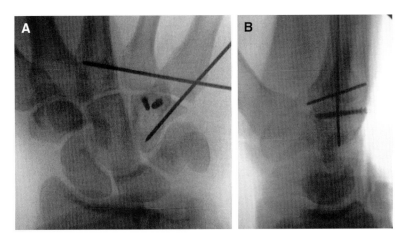

Fig. 2. (*A*) AP and (*B*) lateral radiographs following ORIF of the dorsal hamate fracture with two 2.0-mm screws, reconstruction of the dorsal ligament, and joint reduction and stabilization with two K-wires.

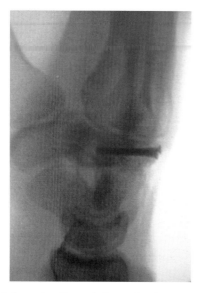

Fig. 3. Lateral radiograph 6 months after reconstruction, showing a healed hamate and a stable fifth CMC joint.

Patients who have missed fracture/dislocations of the finger CMC joints represent the largest group requiring surgical treatment, especially when multiple CMC joints are involved. These injuries are easily overlooked on cursory examination of standard plain radiographs in victims of high-energy trauma, especially by physicians immersed in the care of life threatening injuries. Surgical options include delayed reconstruction by open reduction and internal fixation as well as CMC joint arthrodesis.

Open reduction and internal fixation (ORIF) should be considered in subacute or early chronic cases in which the fracture dislocations involve the fourth and fifth CMC joints, with the goal being maintenance of ulnar column mobility (Fig. 1). Successful ORIF should take place no more than 4 to 6 months following the initial injury, and requires a reconstructable dorsal carpal lip as well as intact cartilaginous surfaces. The technique involves stabilization of the dorsal carpal fracture with screws or Kirschner wires (K-wires), followed by reduction and pinning of the joint and repair of the dorsal ligaments and capsule (Fig. 2). Though there are no large case series, this approach has been effective in the hands of this author and others (Fig. 3) [9,16].

When the radial CMC joints are involved or in chronic cases, concern turns to restoring stability rather than mobility (Figs. 4 and 5). In this situation, arthrodesis is the treatment of choice, and will yield a predictably good result if performed with surgical precision [17]. Typically a cancellous or corticocancellous graft is obtained from the dorsal distal radius, the joint is meticulously decorticated and reduced, then stabilized with a miniplate or K-wires (Fig. 6).

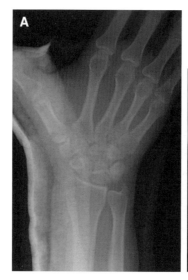
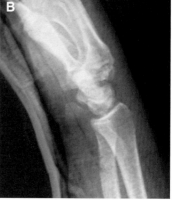

Fig. 4. (A) AP and (B) lateral radiographs revealing missed third and fourth CMC joint fracture dislocations in a severely traumatized patient 6 months following the injury.

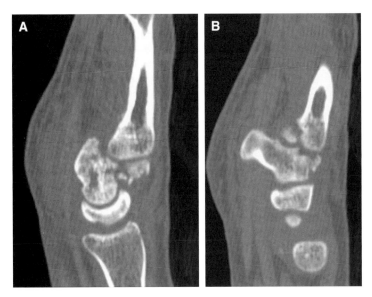

Fig. 5. Sagittal CT scan images detailing the bony destruction of the third (*A*) and fourth (*B*) CMC joints.

Treatment of degenerative arthrosis

Degenerative changes, not related to fracture or dislocation, typically affect the second and third CMC joints, and result in dorsal hypertrophic osteophyte formation. Patients present complaining of a tender prominence over the interval between the two joints. The pain may result strictly from direct pressure or may be related to use and overuse of the digits, sometimes associated with extensor tendon subluxation over the dorsal prominence (Fig. 7). The prominence is firm and nonmobile, consistent with a bony

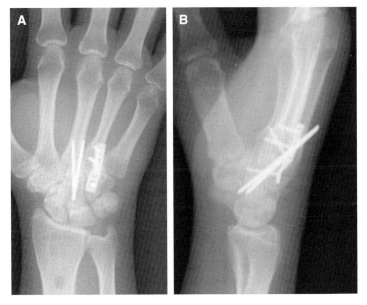

Fig. 6. (*A*) AP and (*B*) lateral radiographs following arthrodesis. The fourth CMC joint is stabilized with a 2.0-mm miniplate. The third CMC joint is stabilized with K-wires. The anatomy of the dorsal capitate did not allow placement of a plate without restricting joint motion.

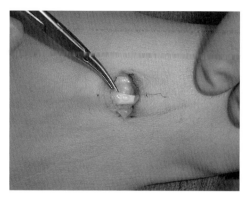

Fig. 7. The bony projection is visualized between the extensor tendons. This patient's symptoms resulted from repeated tendon subluxation and the resulting inflammation.

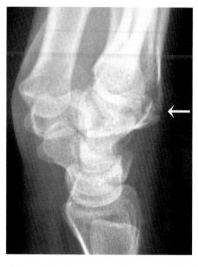

Fig. 9. Even without the "carpal boss view" this lateral radiograph nicely depicts the dorsal third carpometacarpal boss (*arrow*).

mass. It is best visualized clinically with wrist flexion (Fig. 8), and best seen radiographically using a "carpal boss view," with the wrist in 30° of supination and 30° of ulnar deviation (Fig. 9) [18]. The bony mass may be accompanied by mild soft-tissue swelling or a mass characteristic of a ganglion cyst.

In the great majority of cases conservative management suffices. When extensor tendon subluxation is present or a ganglion cyst accompanies the bony prominence, surgery is a more likely possibility. When persistent symptoms exist, the mass is approached through a dorsal transverse incision. If a ganglion cyst is present, it is located

and excised along with its capsular "stalk." The osteophyte is exposed subperiosteally through a longitudinal incision, sometimes requiring limited elevation of the insertion of a radial wrist extensor. An osteotome (Fig. 10) is used to excise the osteophyte from the carpometacarpal joint down to the level of normal joint cartilage (Fig. 11). Palpation ensures complete resection and elimination of tendon subluxation. The dorsal tendon insertion, ligament, and capsule are repaired as required.

Most reports indicate that simple surgical excision of the osteophyte and associated ganglion

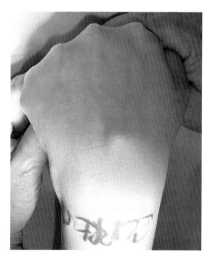

Fig. 8. This dorsal third carpometacarpal boss is best visualized with wrist flexion.

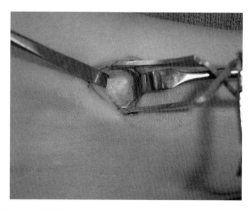

Fig. 10. Following subperiosteal exposure of the dorsal base of the third metacarpal and CMC joint, an osteotome is used to remove the bony projection down to normal articular cartilage.

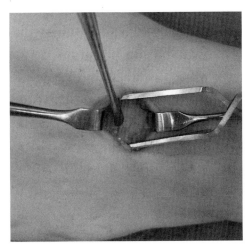

Fig. 11. The elevator is pointing to the third CMC joint following complete boss resection.

provides effective symptom relief in greater than 90% of patients [12,19–21]. Persistent symptoms are thought to be caused by incomplete mass excision [12], regrowth of the bony prominence, or secondary instability. Interestingly, Citteur and coworkers [22] documented instability of the third CMC joint following a standard boss excision performed in cadavers. Passive range of motion at that joint approximately doubled. At surgery, this increased passive motion of the joint is apparent in many patients. It seems plausible that persistent symptoms, not attributable to incomplete excision, may relate to subtle joint instability. Ultimately, CMC joint arthrodesis may be required in such cases.

Summary

Symptomatic post-traumatic arthritis affecting the finger CMC joints is less common than might otherwise be expected based on the frequency of injury, especially to the fifth CMC joint. For the fifth CMC joint, the shallow concavoconvex articulation combined with the typical fracture location may provide a protective effect. Nonoperative measures are typically successful, except in cases of missed fracture/dislocations and symptomatic joint instability. In these instances, reconstruction emphasizes stability first, with an eye toward mobility for the ulnar column.

It is common to detect a bony prominence in the region of the dorsal second and third CMC joints during examination of the hand. In most instances, the projection is asymptomatic and likely represents an os styloideum [18]. When painful and unresponsive to nonoperative treatments, this carpometacarpal boss can be excised surgically.

References

[1] Kraus VB, Li YJ, Martin ER, et al. Articular hypermobility is a protective factor for hand osteoarthritis. Arthritis Rheum 2004;50(7):2178–83.

[2] Nakamura K, Patterson RM, Viegas SF. The ligament and skeletal anatomy of the second through fifth carpometacarpal joints and adjacent structures. J Hand Surg [Am] 2001;26(6):1016–29.

[3] Gunther SF. The carpometacarpal joints. Orthop Clin North Am 1984;15(2):259–77.

[4] El-Shennawy M, Nakamura K, Patterson RM, et al. Three-dimensional kinematic analysis of the second through fifth carpometacarpal joints. J Hand Surg [Am] 2001;26(6):1030–5.

[5] Niechajev I. Dislocated intra-articular fracture of the base of the fifth metacarpal: a clinical study of 23 patients. Plast Reconstr Surg 1985;75(3):406–10.

[6] Yoshida R, Shah MA, Patterson RM, et al. Anatomy and pathomechanics of ring and small finger carpometacarpal joint injuries. J Hand Surg [Am] 2003;28(6):1035–43.

[7] Kjaer-Petersen K, Jurik AG, Petersen LK. Intra-articular fractures at the base of the fifth metacarpal. A clinical and radiographical study of 64 cases. J Hand Surg [Br] 1992;17(2):144–7.

[8] Lundeen JM, Shin AY. Clinical results of intraarticular fractures of the base of the fifth metacarpal treated by closed reduction and cast immobilization. J Hand Surg [Br] 2000;25(3):258–61.

[9] Bora FW Jr, Didizian NH. The treatment of injuries to the carpometacarpal joint of the little finger. J Bone Joint Surg Am 1974;56(7):1459–63.

[10] Pellegrini VD Jr. Fractures at the base of the thumb. Hand Clin 1988;4(1):87–102.

[11] Athanasian EA. Bone and soft tissue tumors. In: Green DP, Hotchkiss RN, Pederson WC, et al, editors. Green's operative hand surgery. Philadelphia: Elsevier; 2005. p. 2211–63.

[12] Fusi S, Watson HK, Cuono CB. The carpal boss. A 20-year review of operative management. J Hand Surg [Br] 1995;20(3):405–8.

[13] Black DM, Watson HK, Vender MI. Arthroplasty of the ulnar carpometacarpal joints. J Hand Surg [Am] 1987;12(6):1071–4.

[14] Green WL, Kilgore ES Jr. Treatment of fifth digit carpometacarpal arthritis with Silastic prosthesis. J Hand Surg [Am] 1981;6(5):510–4.

[15] Gainor BJ, Stark HH, Ashworth CR, et al. Tendon arthroplasty of the fifth carpometacarpal joint for

treatment of posttraumatic arthritis. J Hand Surg [Am] 1991;16(3):520 4.

[16] Imbriglia JE. Chronic dorsal carpometacarpal dislocation of the index, middle, ring, and little fingers. a case report. J Hand Surg [Am] 1979;4(4):343–5.

[17] Clendenin MB, Smith RJ. Fifth metacarpal/hamate arthrodesis for posttraumatic osteoarthritis. J Hand Surg [Am] 1984;9(3):374–8.

[18] Conway WF, Destouet JM, Gilula LA, et al. The carpal boss: an overview of radiographic evaluation. Radiology 1985;156(1):29–31.

[19] Cuono CB, Watson HK. The carpal boss: surgical treatment and etiological considerations. Plast Reconstr Surg 1979;63(1):88–93.

[20] Clarke AM, Wham DJ, Vigvanathan S, et al. The symptomatic carpal boss. Is simple excision enough? J Hand Surg [Br] 1999;24(5):591–5.

[21] Hultgren T, Lugnegard H. Carpal boss. Acta Orthop Scand 1986;57(6):547–50.

[22] Citteur JM, Ritt MJ, Bos KE. Carpal boss: destabilization of the third carpometacarpal joint after a wedge excision. J Hand Surg [Br] 1998;23(1):76–8.

ELSEVIER
SAUNDERS

Hand Clin 22 (2006) 229

HAND
CLINICS

Erratum

In the article "Arthroscopic Techniques for Wrist Arthritis (Radial Styloidectomy and Proximal Pole Hamate Excisions)" by Jeffrey Yao, MD, and A. Lee Osterman, MD, in the November 2005 issue, "Wrist Arthritis," Figs. 6 and 7 were not properly credited to Steven F. Viegas, MD, Professor and Chief, Division of Hand Surgery, Department of Orthopaedic Surgery at the University of Texas Medical Branch in Galveston, Texas. We apologize for this oversight.

ELSEVIER
SAUNDERS

Hand Clin 22 (2006) 231–233

HAND CLINICS

Index

Note: Page numbers of article titles are in **boldface** type.

Changing Your Address?

Make sure your subscription changes too! When you notify us of your new address, you can help make our job easier by including an exact copy of your Clinics label number with your old address (see illustration below.) This number identifies you to our computer system and will speed the processing of your address change. Please be sure this label number accompanies your old address and your corrected address—you can send an old Clinics label with your number on it or just copy it exactly and send it to the address listed below.

We appreciate your help in our attempt to give you continuous coverage. Thank you.

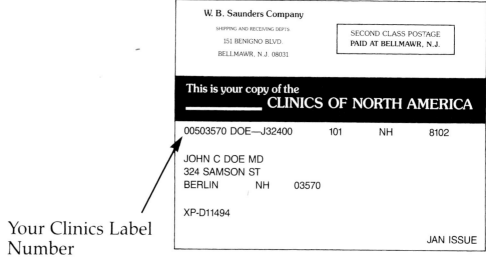

Your Clinics Label Number

Copy it exactly or send your label along with your address to:
Elsevier Periodicals Customer Service
6277 Sea Harbor Drive
Orlando, FL 32887-4800
Call Toll Free 1-800-654-2452

Please allow four to six weeks for delivery of new subscriptions and for processing address changes.